100

DISEASES FOR THE
MRCP PART 2

Commissioning Editor: Laurence Hunter
Project Development Manager: Fiona Conn
Project Manager: Nancy Arnott
Designer: Erik Bigland

100

DISEASES FOR THE
MRCP PART 2

Timothy Gray MA MB BChir, MRCP (London, UK)
Department of Cardiology, Papworth Hospital, Cambridgeshire, UK

Miles Witham BM BCh (Oxon), MRCP (London, UK)
Department of Medicine, Ninewells Hospital, Dundee, UK

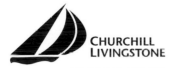

CHURCHILL
LIVINGSTONE

EDINBURGH LONDON NEW YORK PHILADELPHIA ST LOUIS SYDNEY TORONTO 2002

CHURCHILL LIVINGSTONE
An imprint of Harcourt Publishers Limited

© Harcourt Publishers Limited 2002

 is a registered trademark of Harcourt Publishers Limited

The right of Tim Gray and Miles Witham to be identified as
authors of this work has been asserted by them in accordance with
the Copyright, Designs and Patents Act 1988

First published 2002

ISBN 0 443 06466 0

British Library Cataloguing in Publication Data
A catalogue record for this book is available from the British
Library

Library of Congress Cataloging in Publication Data
A catalog record for this book is available from the Library of
Congress

Note
Medical knowledge is constantly changing. As new information
becomes available, changes in treatment, procedures, equipment
and the use of drugs become necessary. The editor, contributors
and the publishers have taken care to ensure that the information
given in this text is accurate and up to date. However, readers are
strongly advised to confirm that the information, especially with
regard to drug usage, complies with the latest legislation and
standards of practice.

The
publisher's
policy is to use
**paper manufactured
from sustainable forests**

Printed in China

PREFACE

Most of the books on the market dealing with the written section of the MRCP part 2 are question based – that is, the information is accessed as the answer to a typical exam question. Whilst we were revising for the exam, we noticed that a number of diseases kept on cropping up in the answers, but we could not find a concise and easily accessible source of information about the symptoms, signs and investigations results for these diseases.

We hope that this book answers that need, and provides a complementary way of learning for the exam. We have included quesions to illustrate how the diseases may present in the exam, and we have tried to codify some of the advice given to us on how to spot probable answers. We hope you find this book useful, not only for the exam, but on the wards after you pass!

We would like to thank all those who helped and supported us in the preparation of this book. Particular mention should go to Justine Davies and Trish Clarke for their longstanding patience and encouragement. Many thanks to Richard Coulden and Emer Sonnex of Papworth Hospital and Rebecca Duell of Southampton Hospital for their help with the X-rays. Thanks also to Sarah Reader and Drew Provan for their support.

We would also like to thank Laurence Hunter and Fiona Conn for their continued and constant support and patience.

Tim Gray
Miles Witham

CONTENTS

CARDIAC DISEASE

1

EISENMENGER'S SYNDROME

Eisenmenger's syndrome occurs when there is significant communication between pulmonary and systemic circulation. The syndrome occurs when the blood flow reverses direction (flow from right to left) due to increased right-sided pressures. The site of the defect is usually divided into pre- and posttricuspid, and this determines the presentation.

Pretricuspid defects (e.g. ASD, single atrium and sinus venosum defects)
The left and right ventricles at birth are the same size and the right ventricle usually regresses with the reduction of right-sided pressures at birth. In pretricuspid defect cases, although there is increased flow (often 3 : 1 +), the right ventricle regresses normally and dilates to accommodate the increased flow and protect the pulmonary vasculature. The shunt by definition bypasses the left ventricle which is usually normal. Eisenmenger's in this situation is unusual, is often atypical, occurs late (90% present in adulthood) and heart failure is rare.

Posttricuspid defects (e.g. VSD, single ventricle and patent ductus arteriosus)
High flow rates (3 : 1–5 : 1) and high pressure from birth in the right ventricle stop the normal right ventricular regression. Pulmonary artery smooth muscular hypertrophy occurs with reduced lung compliance, and increased work of breathing. This causes right ventricular failure and obliterative pulmonary changes. 80% present in infancy.

SYMPTOMS

Dyspnoea, ankle swelling, fatigue, syncope from low output state
Headache, dizziness, visual disturbance from hyperviscosity
Palpitations
Haemoptysis and excessive bleeding
Stroke from hyperviscosity, paradoxical embolus and cerebral abscess

SIGNS

Cyanosis and clubbing (feet only if PDA)
Parasternal heave
Lungs are typically clear

Heart sounds
Loud pulmonary component of second heart sound (sometimes palpable)
Right-sided S4
Single S2 in VSD or wide and fixed in ASD
Pulmonary regurgitation murmur (Graham Steel)
Pulmonary ejection click and murmur
Peripheral oedema if RV failure
NO murmur of VSD or PDA

INVESTIGATIONS

FBC
Hb ↑
Hct ↑
WCC normal
Platelets normal or ↓

U + Es
Urea and creatinine ↑ if congestive cardiac failure

LFTs
Abnormal if congestive cardiac failure

ESR ↓
Clotting normal or prolonged
Urate ↑

ECG
P pulmonale
↑ RV ± LV hypertrophy
Atrial arrhythmias

CXR
↑ PA with oligaemic lung fields – 'pruning'
May see calcification of the PA
Cardiomegaly in ASD but normal heart size typical of VSD/PDA

Angiography
Pressure measurements
Measurement of pulmonary vascular resistance pre- and postvasodilatation with oxygen to look for reversibility

DIAGNOSIS

Echocardiography
Identifies defects and valve abnormalities
Colour mapping may show flow across the shunt
TOE better for visualization of ASD or PDA

DIFFERENTIAL DIAGNOSIS

Primary pulmonary hypertension
Pulmonary vascular obstruction
Pulmonary vascular disease
Lung disease, e.g. restrictive interstitial lung
   disease
Left atrial hypertension
Left ventricular diastolic dysfunction

COMPLICATIONS

Endocarditis
Hyperviscosity and CVAs
Haemostatic abnormalities with reduced clotting
   factors and platelets
Cholelithiasis
Hypertrophic osteoarthropathy
Hyperuricaemia and gout
Renal dysfunction
Haemoptysis

TREATMENT

Avoidance of calcium channel blockers (reduce
   systemic blood pressure and so increase
   shunt), antiplatelet and anticoagulant drugs
   due to increased risk of bleeding
Antibiotic prophylaxis against endocarditis
Isovolaemic phlebotomy (only if symptomatic or
   if Hct > 0.65 with a bleeding diathesis). If
symptoms persist despite phlebotomy then
   consider iron deficiency state
Transplant – heart/lung or lung with repair of
   defect if normal LV function and no coronary
   disease

PROGNOSIS

80% 10 year survival, 77% 15 year and 42%
   25 year
Death mostly due to arrhythmia, also heart
   failure, haemoptysis, brain abscess, embolism
Transplant survival: 70% 1 year, 50% 5 year,
   30% 10 year
Pregnancy mortality 45%, with 50% being
   premature and 40% spontaneous abortion rate
Up to 19% mortality rate with noncardiac
   surgery so best avoided if possible.

QUESTION SPOTTING

Grey case
May occur in this section. New presentation of
Eisenmenger's in an adult is almost always due
to an ASD and is less likely to present with heart
failure, and more likely with arrhythmia or
hyperviscosity syndrome.

Data interpretation
Good for interpretation of cardiac catheter
pressure data.

INFECTIVE ENDOCARDITIS

Microbial infection of the endothelial surface of the heart. This is usually bacterial, but may be fungal or an atypical organism. The disease usually occurs on the heart valves (in order of mitral, aortic, tricuspid and pulmonary) but may also affect septal defects, cardiac tendinae, shunts including patent ductus arteriosus and coarctation. The vegetations consist of fibrin, collagen, platelets, red and white blood cells, and bacteria. These cause destruction of cardiac tissue leading to valvular incompetence, chordae rupture and abscess formation; embolization of vegetation leads to septic foci in distal organs such as CNS, lungs, kidneys and spleen; immune complex vasculitis, especially affecting the kidneys.

Table 1

	Native valve	Prosthetic valve
Streptococcus species	55%	45%
Staphylococcus aureus	7%	11%
Gram negative bacilli	5%	1%
Coagulase negative staphylococci	4%	15%

Most common organisms can be seen in Table 1.

Risk factors
No known predisposing factors in 20–40%. Predisposing factors include rheumatic heart disease, congenital heart disease, mitral valve prolapse with mitral regurgitation, degenerative heart disease, intravenous drug abuse, hypertrophic cardiomyopathy, prosthetic valves and previous endocarditis.

SYMPTOMS
Fever
Sweats
Weight loss
Fatigue
Anorexia
Dyspnoea
Cough
Stroke
Headache
Arthralgia
Chest pain
Confusion

SIGNS
Fever
Murmurs
Tachycardia
Splenomegaly
Clubbing – rare except in prolonged illness
Oedema
Neurological deficit due to abscess or cerebral embolization
Embolic features and immune complex deposition: splinter haemorrhages, petechiae, Janeway lesions, Roth spots and Osler's nodes

INVESTIGATIONS

FBC
Hb ↓ (normochromic, normocytic)
WCC ↑
Platelets normal

U + Es
Urea and creatinine may be ↑

LFTs
Albumin ↓
Immunoglobulins ↑
Otherwise usually normal

ESR ↑
CRP ↑
Clotting normal
False positive VDRL
Complement levels ↓

Urine
Proteinuria and haematuria in 50%

CXR
Cardiomegaly
Pulmonary congestion
Cannon ball lesions seen with right-sided endocarditis from septic emboli

ECG
↑ PR interval if aortic root involvement

DIAGNOSIS

Dukes criteria

Major
1) Positive blood cultures – organism grown from two separate cultures or persistent positive cultures 12 h apart

2) Evidence of endocardial involvement, i.e. echocardiographic evidence of vegetation, abscess or new dehiscence, or new valve murmur

Minor
Predisposition to endocarditis
Fever >38°C
Vascular or immunogenic phenomena, e.g. splinter haemorrhages
Positive blood cultures (non-major)
Positive ECHO (non-major), e.g. valve incompetence

Diagnosis depends on 2 major, 1 major and 3 minor or 5 minor
Blood cultures × 3 positive in 90%
Serology for aspergillus, candida, Q fever, chlamydia, brucella if appropriate
CO_2 culture for HACEK organisms if otherwise culture negative

Echocardiography
Transthoracic sensitive in 58–63% in native valve endocarditis but less if prosthetic
Transoesophageal echocardiography sensitive in 90–100%

COMPLICATIONS

Embolic
Cerebral, renal, splenic, hepatic infarcts and mycotic aneurysms if left-sided endocarditis
Pulmonary infarcts or abscesses if right-sided endocarditis

Cardiac
Valvular failure, unstable prosthesis, fistula formation, abscess formation, AV nodal block and valvular obstruction if vegetation enlarges

Renal
Vasculitis

TREATMENT

Antibiotic therapy
Prolonged intravenous antibiotics (usually 4–12 weeks). Frequently benzylpenicillin and gentamycin for 2 weeks followed by oral amoxycillin for 4 weeks if penicillin sensitive

Streptococcus. Follow British National Formulary guidelines. Doses dependent on MIC and MBC (minimum inhibitory concentration and minimum bacteriocidal concentration). Length of treatment depends on organism isolated.

If culture negative with native valve endocarditis, give ampicillin and gentamycin. If prosthetic valve and culture negative, add in vancomycin.

Surgery
Absolute indications
Uncontrolled infection
Relapse after therapy with prosthetic valve
Unstable prosthesis
Moderate to severe heart failure due to valve dysfunction

Relative indications
Relapse after therapy with native valve
Perivalvular extension of infection
Large vegetations
Staphylococcus aureus infection or fungal infection
Culture negative endocarditis with persistent fever

Prevention
Prophylactic antibiotics prior to:
Dental work involving work below the gum line
Surgical procedures, especially if any pre-existing infection
Cystoscopy and urinary tract instrumentation
Prostatic biopsy
Pacemaker insertion
Rigid bronchoscopy (but not flexible)
Vaginal delivery if infection present
Colonoscopy and biopsy especially if inflammation

Patients who need prophylaxis include those with:

Prosthetic heart valves
Previous infective endocarditis
Congenital heart disease including PDA, VSD, coarctation
Valvular pathology
Surgically corrected anomalies
Hypertrophic cardiomyopathy

QUESTION SPOTTING

Grey case

Endocarditis is a multisystem disorder that has a long differential diagnosis (*see* SLE). Because of the serious nature of the disease, it is essential to consider it in any patient presenting with a murmur and fever. CRP is a better marker than ESR for active disease, cf. SLE.

Data interpretation

Less likely to crop up in this section.

Rheumatic fever is a systemic connective tissue disease occurring approximately 3 weeks after a group A streptococcal infection. It causes inflammation of the heart, central nervous system and joints, probably due to cross reactivity of the streptococcal M protein with cardiac and other organ tissue which leads to an autoimmune reaction. This leads to the pathognomonic Aschoff lesion which is collagen degeneration associated with infiltration of mononuclear cells and multinucleated histiocytes. The disease typically affects 6–16 year olds, who often have genetic predisposition.

CLINICAL FEATURES

The diagnosis is clinical and defined by the Duckett Jones criteria:

Major criteria

Pancarditis (>50%)
Endocarditis: Valvulitis most frequently involving mitral and aortic valves causing valvular insufficiency and scarring. Murmurs are common, including a non-specific mid systolic murmur, the Carey Coombes murmur (mid-diastolic murmur of thickened mitral valves). Nodules may form on the valve leaflets.
    Myocarditis: causes cardiac failure, conduction defects and arrhythmias.
    Pericarditis: pericardial effusion, friction rub and chest pains.

Polyarthritis (60%)
Typically an asymmetrical, large joint migratory polyarthritis. The arthritis tends to be more prominent than carditis in adults and vice versa in children.

Chorea (20%)
Sydenham's chorea, St Vitus' dance
May be the only clinical finding. May include emotional lability and explosive speech.

Erythema marginatum (5%)

Subcutaneous nodules (5%)

Minor criteria
Arthralgia
Fever
↑ ESR/CRP
↑ PR interval

Previous rheumatic fever
Leucocytosis

Two minor, or one major plus two minor, criteria are necessary for diagnosis. Plus supporting evidence of preceding group A streptococcal infection by throat swab culture, ↑ ASOT or other streptococcal antibody test.

INVESTIGATIONS

FBC
Hb ↓ (MCV normal)
WCC ↑ though variable. Neutrophilia
Platelets normal
ESR ↑

U + Es
Usually normal

LFTs
Albumin normal or ↓
Otherwise normal

CRP ↑
CK ↑
Troponins ↑
↑ ASOT titre and levels >200 units

CXR
Cardiomegaly
Increased pulmonary vascular markings
Pulmonary oedema

ECG
PR interval ↑
Tachycardia
AV block
Non-specific QRS and T wave changes

Echocardiogram
Cardiac dilatation
Valvular abnormalities
Pericardial effusion

DIAGNOSIS

Clinical diagnosis based on Duckett Jones criteria and echocardiographic findings

DIFFERENTIAL DIAGNOSIS

SLE
Acute juvenile arthritis or Still's disease

Infective endocarditis
Pericarditis
Viral illness with arthralgia

TREATMENT

Bed rest until inflammatory markers are normal.
   Penicillin for 10 days to treat streptococcal
infection (erythromycin in penicillin
hypersensitivity).
   Aspirin (60 mg/kg/day) in divided doses for at
least a month in mild carditis or arthritis.
   Prednisolone 1–2 mg/kg/day for 2–3 months if
severe cardiac disease.
   Rebound carditis and arthritis is often seen on
weaning off steroids, and aspirin is indicated for
this.
   Valve replacement if acute severe valvular
insufficiency.

Primary prevention
Penicillin as early as possible in streptococcal
pharyngitis.

Secondary prevention
Continuous penicillin for 5 years or until
21 years of age (whichever is longer) if no
carditis. May be needed for longer and
sometimes life if carditis.

PROGNOSIS

There is a recurrence rate of 50% in patients who
have previously had the disease who then get a
group A streptococcal pharyngitis.

QUESTION SPOTTING

Grey case
Watch for the Duckett Jones criteria and be
especially alerted if chorea is present.
Pericarditis is commoner than endocarditis in
rheumatic fever.

Data interpretation
Less suited for this type of question.

EBSTEIN'S ANOMALY

Downward displacement of the septal and inferior leaflets of tricuspid valve. The upper portion of the right ventricle becomes atrialized leading to a small right ventricle. The valve leaflets are often abnormal and may adhere to the right ventricular wall leading to a variable degree of tricuspid regurgitation. There is also a variable degree of right ventricular outflow obstruction (pulmonary atresia or stenosis) in 30%.

Maternal exposure to lithium in the first trimester has been implicated.

SYMPTOMS

Dyspnoea
Palpitations

SIGNS

Cyanosis
Clubbing possible
Signs of TR: pansystolic murmur, giant V wave of JVP, pulsatile liver, systolic thrill
Wide splitting of S1 and S2 ± S3 ± S4

INVESTIGATIONS

ECG
RBBB
WPW Type B – delta waves, short PR interval and predominantly negative deflection in V1 and V2
P pulmonale
↑ PR interval
Wide QRS

CXR
Enlarged right atrium
Oligaemic lung fields

Cardiac catheter
Atrial pressure with right ventricular complexes in the right ventricle

DIAGNOSIS

Echocardiography
Low tricuspid valve
Late valve closure
Abnormal anterior valve cusp

ASSOCIATIONS

ASD secundum 50%
pSVT/AF 25%
Pulmonary stenosis/atresia 30%
Wolff-Parkinson-White Type B 10%
ASD primum rare
VSD rare

DIFFERENTIAL DIAGNOSIS

Right ventricular dysplasia
Pulmonary stenosis
Dilated cardiomyopathy

TREATMENT

Systemic pulmonary shunt and later Fontan procedure.

Reconstruction of the tricuspid valve, ASD closure, tricuspid annuloplasty and plication of atrialized right ventricle

If pre-excitation, cardiac radiofrequency ablation or surgical division.

QUESTION SPOTTING

Grey case
Watch out for patients presenting with signs of right heart failure and tricuspid regurgitation in conjunction with palpitations from WPW. Likewise watch out for ASD with WPW which may indicate Ebstein's anomaly.

Data interpretation
May crop up in this section with some angiogram pressure and saturation data.

ATRIAL SEPTAL DEFECTS

The true atrial septal defects are those that originate from the fossa ovalis giving rise to ostium secundum defects. However the term is also often used to include any communication between left and right sides of the heart at atrial level. These lesions include ostium primum defects, sinus venosus defects, inferior vena cava defects and coronary sinus anomalies.

The male : female ratio is 1 : 4. Ostium primum defects tend to present in childhood. Ostium secundum defects often present in adulthood and often with atrial fibrillation.

SYMPTOMS

Usually asymptomatic in early years
Fatigue
Exertional dyspnoea
Chest infections
Palpitations

SIGNS

Irregular pulse
↑ JVP
Right ventricular heave
S1 normal or split, S2 wide fixed split
Mid systolic ejection flow murmur
Mid diastolic tricuspid flow murmur
Pansystolic murmur of mitral regurgitation if associated mitral valve abnormalities including MV prolapse

INVESTIGATIONS

ECG

Primum: RVH, RBBB, right axis deviation
Secundum: RVH, RBBB, left axis deviation
Sinus venosus: RVH, RBBB, right axis deviation, left axis P waves
May have ↑ PR interval

CXR

Large RA and RV
Large PA and pulmonary markings

DIAGNOSIS

Echocardiography

Large RA, RV and PA
Mitral valve abnormalities
Direct visualization of the defect

Cardiac catheter

Useful to work out shunting with saturation measurements
Catheter may pass through defect and may identify other defects
Right-sided pressures often normal unless pulmonary hypertension

ASSOCIATIONS

Down's syndrome

DIFFERENTIAL DIAGNOSIS

VSD
PDA
Endocardial cushion defect

COMPLICATIONS

Infective endocarditis in ostium primum defects
Pulmonary hypertension (15%) as late complication
Eisenmenger's syndrome (6–9%)
Cardiac failure
Atrial arrhythmias
Paradoxical embolus

TREATMENT

Antibiotic prophylaxis for dental work.
Surgical closure if uncomplicated ASD with significant shunt (>1.5 : 1). This is best performed in children aged 2–5 and has a mortality of <1%.
Percutaneous closure now possible with deployable dumb-bell devices but these have limitations.

QUESTION SPOTTING

Grey case

May be part of an Eisenmenger's complex or be the cause of infective endocarditis.

Data interpretation

Most likely to come up as cardiac catheterization data. Remember that in ASDs the ventricular saturations will be the same, whereas in VSDs the left ventricular saturations may be different from aortic saturations.

CARDIAC MYXOMAS

Tumours of mesenchymal origin, occurring in the heart. Although they tend not to be invasive, embolization is common. The cause is not clearly established, but some tumours show cytogenetic abnormalities, especially in cases of Carney's syndrome (see below). 86% are in the left atrium, and usually arise from the septal wall, and 90% are solitary. Less commonly they arise in the right atrium and rarely in the ventricles. 10% of cases are familial and probably autosomal dominant.

SYMPTOMS

Fever
Weight loss
Exertional dyspnoea
Paroxysmal dyspnoea
Syncope
Haemoptysis
Some symptoms may vary with body position
Also arthralgia, myalgia, chest pain
Stroke

SIGNS

Irregular pulse
Clubbing
Raynaud's phenomenon
Mid diastolic murmur of mitral stenosis which may vary with position
Pansystolic murmur of mitral regurgitation
Loud P2 and right heart failure if right-sided
Tumour 'plop'

INVESTIGATIONS

FBC
Hb ↓ (MCV normal)
WCC ↑
Platelets normal or rarely ↓
ESR ↑
Clotting normal

U + Es
Urea and creatinine ↑ if renal vasculitis or embolization

LFTs
Globulins ↑
Albumin ↓

CRP ↑

Urinalysis
Blood and protein if renal vasculitis or embolization

DIAGNOSIS

Echocardiography
Allows accurate estimation of size, position and mobility of the tumour. May be difficult to differentiate from atrial thrombus

Transoesophageal echocardiography (TOE)
Often superior to transthoracic echocardiography

Cardiac catheter
Has risk of tumour embolization, but should be performed if there is suspicion of underlying coronary artery disease

ASSOCIATIONS

A few cases are as part of the 'syndrome myxoma' or 'Carney's syndrome': cardiac myxoma (may be multiple, recurrent after surgery, and more often in other chambers of the heart)
Myxomas in other sites, e.g. skin
Freckled pigmentation of the skin
Endocrine tumours, e.g. pituitary, testicular, adrenal cortex

DIFFERENTIAL DIAGNOSIS

Connective tissue diseases
Infective endocarditis
Atrial thrombus
Rheumatic fever
Other occult malignancy

COMPLICATIONS

Embolization to brain, lung and peripheral vessels which may show malignant tendencies with local invasion and destruction giving rise to myxomatous pseudoaneurysms.

TREATMENT

Urgent surgical resection. Low mortality rates reported (2%)

Recurrence is in the order of 1–5% following resection (up to 22% if familial type)

QUESTION SPOTTING

Grey case

Atrial myxoma may mimic connective tissue diseases but appropriate testing with ANA, ANCA, rheumatoid factor etc. should help. If echocardiography suggests an intracardiac mass, or clinical examination suggests a new murmur, then infective endocarditis is clearly an important diagnosis to rule out. Blood cultures should be the investigation of choice in this situation.

Data interpretation

Unlikely to appear in this section.

RESPIRATORY DISEASE

2

SARCOIDOSIS

Sarcoidosis is a multisystem disorder of unknown aetiology. The hallmark of the disease is the presence of non-caseating granulomas in affected organ systems. Almost any organ system may be involved, making it the ideal MRCP topic. Afro-Caribbeans are affected more commonly. Peak age of onset 25–40 years.

CLINICAL FEATURES

May be asymptomatic

Constitutional
Fever
Malaise
Weight loss
Peripheral lymphadenopathy

Respiratory
Dry cough (>90%)
SOB on exertion
Wheeze
Crackles occur only when fibrosis is established
Clubbing is rare
Pleural effusion (uncommon)

Skin/joints
Arthralgia (12–27%)
Acute polyarthropathy may also occur, especially at the onset of the illness
Bone pain (cysts – 5%)
Tendon and joint inflammation
Lupus pernio
Violaceous plaques
Maculopapular rash
Subcutaneous nodules
Erythema nodosum

Eyes
Painful eyes – anterior uveitis
Blurred vision (uveitis, papilloedema, chorioretinitis)
Dry eyes (lacrimitis)
Band keratopathy (from hypercalcaemia)

Neurological
Meningism (5%)
Cranial nerve palsies (esp. VIIn – may be bilateral)
Thirst, polyuria (hypothalamic involvement or hypercalcaemia)
Seizures
Psychosis
Paraesthesia and focal weakness (peripheral neuropathy, transverse myelitis)

Cardiac
Sudden death (heart block, arrhythmias)
Cardiomyopathy
Ventricular aneurysm – very rare

Other
Dry mouth (parotitis)
Hepatomegaly (25%, usually asymptomatic, but may give rise to portal hypertension and varices)
Splenomegaly (25%)

INVESTIGATIONS

FBC
Usually normal
Lymphocytes may be $\downarrow$
Hb, WCC and platelets $\downarrow$ if spleen enlarged

U + Es
Usually normal

LFTs
Calcium – may be $\uparrow$
Bilirubin, ALP mildly $\uparrow$ if liver involved
Albumin may be $\downarrow$

ESR often $\uparrow$
CRP usually normal
Immunoglobulins may be $\uparrow$
Serum ACE – $\uparrow$ in two-thirds (>2 SD above normal)

Urinary calcium often $\uparrow$

Chest X-ray
Bilateral hilar LNs in 90% in acute disease
May show midzone or diffuse fibrosis. See example chest X-ray (Fig. 1)

Abdominal X-ray
May show nephrocalcinosis

ECG
May show AV block or conduction delay

PFTs
Reduced FVC and TLco. FEV_1 may also be reduced due to obstructive lesions

Tuberculin test negative in two-thirds. A strongly positive test is unusual

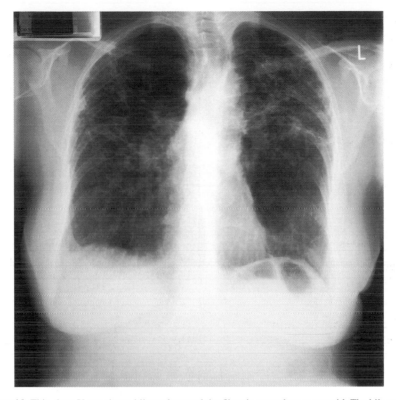

Fig. 1.   Sarcoid. This chest X-ray shows bilateral upper lobe fibrosis secondary to sarcoid. The hila are pulled up and the lower lobes are pulled up and stretched so that tenting can be seen at the diaphragm. There are also cystic changes in the upper lobes.

DIAGNOSIS

Biopsy of lung or skin lesions or other affected organ is usually the most accessible way of diagnosing sarcoid. Lung biopsy reveals the diagnosis in 80% of cases. Diagnosis is by a combination of clinical findings and biopsy result.

The Kveim-Silzbach test is not usually used. Serum ACE level is not specific or sensitive for sarcoidosis, but useful in monitoring disease activity.

DIFFERENTIAL DIAGNOSIS

Sarcoid can mimic many other diseases, as its
  manifestations are so diverse

Lung diseases which may mimic the fibrosis of sarcoid include

Fibrosing alveolitis
Extrinsic allergic alveolitis
Berylliosis (also shows granulomas)
Histiocytosis X

Differential diagnosis for BHL

Tuberculosis
Lymphoma
Metastatic Ca
Histoplasmosis
Coccidiomycosis

COMPLICATIONS

Progressive fibrosis and lung damage can lead to bronchiectasis and aspergillus colonization. Fibrosis also leads to cor pulmonale.

Sudden death or cardiac failure occur secondary to cardiac involvement.

TREATMENT

Indications for steroid therapy include

Neurological disease
Cardiac disease
Eye involvement
Hypercalcaemia
Progressive lung fibrosis
Persistent erythema nodosum

Chloroquine and derivatives can be used as steroid sparing agents.

PROGNOSIS

Lofgrens syndrome (erythema nodosum plus BHL) – 90% remit

BHL alone (50%) – 80% remit within 1 year
BHL and fibrosis (25%) – 50% remit
Fibrosis alone (10%) – 25% remit

QUESTION SPOTTING

Grey case

Sarcoidosis can be used in many different ways but, often, a clue is the combination of respiratory symptoms together with thirst and polyuria. Any cranial nerve lesion, especially if bilateral, should cause suspicion of sarcoid with a differential diagnosis of Lyme disease.

Data interpretation

Questions may depict a patient with shortness of breath, a restrictive defect and a high calcium.

CYSTIC FIBROSIS

A defect in the cystic fibrosis transmembrane conductance regulator gene (CFTR) located on the long arm of chromosome 7 is thought to be the cause of most cases. This gene is essential for the regulation of salt and water movement across cell membranes. The gene represents a transmembrane chloride channel, and a defect leads to an alteration in shape and thus a failure to open in response to elevated cAMP. This causes failure of excretion of chloride and so there is an increased reabsorption of sodium into the epithelial cells. With less salt there is less excretion of water and so the viscosity of mucus produced at the epithelial surface rises. The CFTR is also required for excretion of sweat and CF patients have impaired reabsorption of sodium chloride in the sweat ducts leading to excessive loss of this in sweat.

The most common gene defect is the $\Delta 508$ mutation. This accounts for 70% of cases in the UK and USA. In Southern Europe, this falls to <50% and only 30% in Ashkenazi families. Cystic fibrosis is one of the most common hereditary diseases in Caucasians with a carrier frequency of 1 : 25 and an incidence of about 1 : 2500 live births.

CLINICAL FEATURES

Respiratory
Nasal polyps
Haemoptysis
Recurrent bronchial infections, especially with
   Staphylococcus aureus, *Pseudomonas aeruginosa*, or *Burkholderia cepacia*.
Bronchiectasis from recurrent infections
Spontaneous pneumothorax
Cor pulmonale
Allergic bronchopulmonary aspergillosis

Gastrointestinal
Abdominal pain from:

Pancreatic inflammation and failure leading to steatorrhoea and impaired glucose tolerance
Small bowel obstruction (meconium ileus equivalent)
Biliary cirrhosis and portal hypertension from chronic cholestatic liver disease
Gallstones

Pericholangitis
Periportal hepatic fibrosis

Other
Neurological deficits from vitamin E deficiency (rare)
Clotting abnormalities from vitamin K deficiency (rare)
Male infertility
Secondary amenorrhoea
Amyloid
Arthropathy
Finger clubbing in chronic suppurative lung disease

Infants
Meconium ileus
Failure to thrive
Oedema from hypoalbuminaemia

INVESTIGATIONS

FBC
Hb normal
WCC ↑ if infection
Platelets normal or ↓ if splenomegaly

U + Es
Normal

LFTs
Usually abnormal
Albumin ↓
Immunoglobulins normal
Bilirubin often ↑
AST often ↑
ALP often ↑
Ca may be normal or ↓
Amylase ↓
Glucose ↑ (impaired glucose tolerance)

Pancreatic exocrine function test such as the Lundh test shows impaired exocrine function

CXR
Pneumonia
Bronchiectasis
Pneumothorax
Fibrosis

AXR
Obstruction

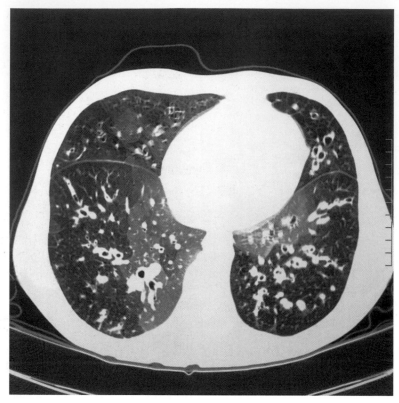

Fig. 2. **Bronchiectasis.** Widespread airway enlargement with air trapping. Patches of lung tissue show higher attenuation. These are normal and reduce in size on expiration. Other areas show low attenuation which are unaltered on expiration; these are areas of alveolitis with air trapping.

See CT Chest – bronchiectasis with air trapping (Fig. 2)

Sputum microscopy and culture for bacterial growth

DIAGNOSIS

High sweat sodium concentration of over 60 mmol/L. Sweat is best elicited by pilocarpine iontophoresis. The sample must be >100 mg.

Immunoreactive trypsin >80 mcg/L in infants of 1–2 weeks, but rapidly falls to below normal after this.

DIFFERENTIAL DIAGNOSIS

Coeliac disease (may co-exist with cystic fibrosis). Look for evidence of villous atrophy.

Congenital pancreatic hypoplasia
Crohn's disease/ulcerative colitis

Causes of bronchiectasis

Postinfectious; measles, rubella, tuberculosis
Allergic bronchopulmonary aspergillosis
Gamma globulin deficiencies
Ciliary immotility, e.g. Kartagener's syndrome
Neuropathic causes such as Chagas' disease and the Riley-Day syndrome which cause autonomic disturbance leading to hypersecretion of mucus
Bronchial obstruction with tumour or foreign body
Idiopathic

TREATMENT

Pancreatic supplements

Chest physiotherapy for sputum production
Antibiotics directed at specific chest pathogens.
  Once colonized with *Pseudomonas* species,
  clearance is rare, but control can be
  maintained with IV antibiotics, via an
  indwelling central venous port. Nebulized
  antibiotics also have a role.
Bronchospasm may be treated with
  bronchodilators.
Genetic counselling.

Other treatments include:
  Nebulized recombinant human DNAase which
breaks down the DNA in inflammatory cells
which is thought to add to the viscosity of the
mucus. This has been shown to improve
FEV_1.
  Nebulized α1-antitrypsin can reduce the
elastase load in neutrophils and improve lung
function.
  Organ transplantation may be considered in
end stage disease.
  Somatic gene therapy by inhaling the normal
CFTR gene in a vector is possible but tissue

uptake is poor and improvement is not
sustained. This remains experimental.

PROGNOSIS

90% survive into their teens.
  Median survival for cystic fibrosis patients
born now is as good as 40 years.

QUESTION SPOTTING

Grey case
Think of CF in the young patient with
malabsorption or recurrent infections. Exclude
hypogammaglobulinaemia which may present
with recurrent respiratory infections and
diarrhoea.

Data interpretation
You may be asked to interpret the results of a
pancreatic stimulation test, but cystic fibrosis is
better suited for the grey case.

BRONCHIAL CARCINOMA

There are 36 000 deaths per year from lung cancer in the UK. This represents 25% of all cancer deaths. Male to female ratio is 3.5 : 1. Cigarette smoking is thought to be responsible for 90% of lung cancers. Passive smoking may cause as much as 5%. Other factors implicated include asbestos, arsenic, chromium, iron oxide, petrol products, tar, coal, silicon, radiation and other causes of alveolitis such as cryptogenic fibrosing alveolitis and systemic sclerosis.

TYPES

Squamous cell carcinoma (35–40%)
Characteristically cavitate and metastasize late.

Adenocarcinoma (10–30%)
Originate from mucus glands, and lead to a subpleural mass. Pleural invasion is common, as are mediastinal lymph nodes. Metastases tend to go to brain and bones. Less association with smoking and more with asbestos.

Small cell carcinoma (Oat cell) (20–50%)
Develop from endocrine Kutchitsky cells (APUD cells). Usually metastatic at presentation. 10% produce ectopic hormones. Only type to have a significant response to chemotherapy.

Large cell carcinoma (15–25%)
Tend to be poorly differentiated and metastasize early.

Alveolar cell carcinoma (1–2%)
Peripheral solitary nodule or diffuse nodular lesions. Usually present with profuse mucoid sputum production.

SYMPTOMS

Weight loss
Anorexia
Lethargy
Cough (40%). Sputum production, especially if bronchial obstruction leads to recurrent pneumonia
Chest pain (20%) from pleural involvement or nerve invasion
Pancoast syndrome is pain in shoulder and inner aspect of arm from lower brachial plexus involvement (especially the T1 nerve root) and associated Horner's syndrome
Haemoptysis particularly if the carcinoma is proximal and endobronchial
Dyspnoea if collapse, bronchial obstruction or lymphangitis
Dysphagia if mediastinal spread
Hoarseness/'bovine' cough if recurrent laryngeal nerve involvement

Symptoms of metastatic spread
Neuro: focal neurological deficit, seizures, personality change
Bones: pain, pathological fractures
Liver: jaundice, abdominal pain
Skin: nodules

Symptoms of non-metastatic disease
Symptoms of hypercalcaemia
Paraneoplastic syndromes

SIGNS

Often normal
Lymphadenopathy, e.g. supraclavicular nodes especially in squamous cell carcinoma
Signs of pneumonia – collapse, consolidation
Stridor
Monophonic unilateral wheeze
Hoarse voice
Dull lung base from phrenic nerve palsy
Pleural effusion
Superior vena cava obstruction
Clubbing ± hypertrophic pulmonary osteoarthropathy

PARANEOPLASTIC SYNDROMES

Endocrine (10%)
SIADH (esp. small cell)
Ectopic ACTH secretion (esp. small cell)
Hypercalcaemia secondary to PTHrP secretion (esp. squamous cell lung carcinoma)
Carcinoid-like syndrome
Gynaecomastia
Thyrotoxicosis
Hypoglycaemia
Addison's disease (due to adrenal replacement with mets)

Neurology
Polyneuropathy

Myelopathy (leading to motor neurone like disease)

Encephalopathy including cerebellar degeneration

Myasthenia (Eaton-Lambert syndrome)

Polymyopathy

Skin
Dermatomyositis
Acanthosis nigricans
Herpes zoster
Erythema gyratum repens

Vascular
Thrombophlebitis migrans
Non-bacterial thrombotic endocarditis
Disseminated intravascular coagulation
Thrombotic thrombocytopenic purpura
Anaemia (normocytic, microcytic, haemolytic)

Other
Clubbing (30%) esp. in adenocarcinoma and squamous cell carcinoma.

Hypertrophic pulmonary osteoarthropathy (3%). May be associated with gynaecomastia (esp. squamous cell and adenocarcinoma).

Eosinophilia

INVESTIGATIONS

FBC
Hb ↓ or normal
WCC normal or ↑ if co-existent infection
Platelets normal

U + Es
Na normal or ↓ if SIADH
K normal or ↓↓ if ectopic ACTH
Urea and creatinine normal

LFTs
Albumin ↓
Ca ↑ if PTHrP secretion
Deranged if liver metastases
Clotting normal

Chest X-ray – 90% sensitive at presentation
Hilar enlargement (unilateral or bilateral)

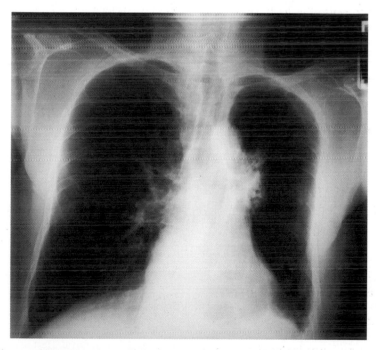

Fig. 3. Carcinoma of lung. This chest radiograph shows a left hilar mass. There is loss of lung volume in the left hemithorax from previous lobectomy and there are pathological rib fractures on the left side.

Peripheral opacity especially with
  adenocarcinoma or alveolar cell carcinoma
Collapse
Effusion
Rib destruction
Pericardial effusion
Lymphangitis carcinomatosa
See chest X-ray (Fig. 3)

DIAGNOSIS

Bronchoscopy and biopsy/bronchial brushings
  (80% within reach of scope)
Sputum cytology
Percutaneous needle biopsy (CT guidance or at
  mediastinoscopy)
Biopsy of possible metastases (lymph node, liver
  or bone marrow)
CT scan of chest (and head/liver for staging)
Liver ultrasound scan
Bone scan
Bone marrow biopsy

DIFFERENTIAL DIAGNOSIS

For haemoptysis
Infection including tuberculosis
Pulmonary embolus
Bronchiectasis
Goodpasture's syndrome
Wegener's granulomatosis
Microscopic polyarteritis
Allergic bronchopulmonary aspergillosis
Idiopathic pulmonary haemosiderosis
Trauma
Benign tumours
Hereditary haemorrhagic telangiectasia
  (Osler-Weber-Rendu)

For round lesions on a chest X-ray
Carcinoma
Secondary tumours
Lung abscess
Encysted interlobar effusion
Hydatid cyst
A–V malformation
Bronchial carcinoid
Aspergilloma
Rheumatoid nodule

Hamartoma
Bronchogenic cyst

For cavitating lesions on a chest X-ray
Infection – *Staphylococcus aureus*, tuberculosis,
  Klebsiella, *Pneumocystis carinii*, hydatid,
  amoebic, fungal
Tumour, esp. squamous cell
Infarcts
Wegener's granulomatosis
Rheumatoid nodules

TREATMENT

Surgical
85% not resectable
Careful staging essential

Contraindications to surgery
Metastases
Mediastinal organ invasion
Malignant pleural effusion
Contralateral mediastinal nodes
FEV_1 <0.8 L
Severe cardiac/other condition

Radiotherapy
Radical especially in conjunction with
  chemotherapy
Palliative for SVCO, haemoptysis, chest
  pain/metastatic pain and major airway
  obstruction.
Watch for radiation pneumonitis (early) and
  radiation fibrosis (late).

Combined chemotherapy
Useful in small cell carcinoma

Laser therapy via fibreoptic bronchoscopy for
  palliating airway obstruction

Also think of:

Bronchial stenting
Steroids
Demeclocycline for SIADH
Palliative care

PROGNOSIS

80% 1 year mortality
Only 6% 5 year survival. Best results are for well
  differentiated squamous cell carcinoma.

QUESTION SPOTTING

Grey case

Remember rarer presentations of common conditions. Bronchial carcinoma is more common than Goodpasture's syndrome as a cause of haemoptysis. Abnormal blood tests may be caused by metastases or paraneoplastic phenomena.

LEGIONELLA PNEUMONIA

Legionella pneumophila is a fastidious gram negative aerobic bacillus, found in cooling towers, showers and other water carrying systems. The organism is spread via aerosols. Between 2% and 15% of community acquired pneumonia is due to *Legionella* in Europe.

SYMPTOMS

Dry cough, becoming purulent later
SOB
Headache
Fever and rigors
Myalgia
Nausea and vomiting
Diarrhoea and abdominal pain (in 20–40%)
Chest pain (may not be pleuritic)

SIGNS

Tachypnoea
Acute confusion
Crackles; sometimes bilateral
Pleural effusion (30%) but usually subclinical
Bronchial breathing (16%)

Less common features
Myocarditis
Pericarditis
Pancreatitis
Pyelonephritis
Peritonitis
Focal neurological signs, e.g. cerebellar dysfunction.

INVESTIGATIONS

FBC
Hb usually normal
WCC normal or mildly ↑, but lymphocytes often ↓
Platelets usually normal

U + Es
Na ↓
K usually normal
Urea often ↑
Creatinine sometimes ↑

LFTs
Abnormal in 50%

ALT ↑
ALP ↑
Bilirubin ↑ in 20%

CK occasionally ↑

Haematuria and proteinuria may be present, as with other forms of pneumonia.

CXR
Shows unilateral lobar shadowing, sometimes multilobar shadowing. Cavitation is rare, and tends to occur in immunosuppressed patients. Small pleural effusion in one-third of cases.

DIAGNOSIS

Culture of sputum (80–90% sensitive)
Sputum fluorescent antibody staining (25–75% sensitive)
Urinary antigen test: sensitivity 70%, specificity 99% for serogroup 1
Fourfold rise in legionella serology during convalescence to a titre of 1 : 64 or greater (75% sensitive)

DIFFERENTIAL DIAGNOSIS

Other atypical pneumonias, e.g.
Mycoplasma
Psittacosis
Q fever

TREATMENT

Macrolides, e.g. erythromycin
Tetracyclines
Quinolones, e.g. ciprofloxacin

Add rifampicin if severely ill

PROGNOSIS

5–15% mortality overall; 75% mortality in immunosuppressed patients.
    20% of patients admitted to hospital will require mechanical ventilation.

QUESTION SPOTTING

Grey case
Consider the diagnosis if:
Foreign travel – especially if air conditioning in old or Third World hotel.

Non-lobar pneumonia
Diarrhoeal prodrome
Failure to respond to penicillins
Deranged LFTs or low sodium (although not
   confined to atypical pneumonias)

Data interpretation
Unlikely to crop up in this section.

MYCOPLASMA PNEUMONIA

Infection by *Mycoplasma pneumoniae*. Many of the extrapulmonary manifestations are thought to be due to a hyperreactive immune response against the organism. Disease is often mild, and may be subclinical. Accounts for up to 15% of pneumonia during epidemic seasons, which occur every 4 to 7 years. Late summer/autumn is peak time of year. Incubation is 2 to 3 weeks.

SYMPTOMS

Prodrome of malaise and headache often precedes chest symptoms by 1 to 5 days.

Cough – usually non-productive
SOB
Nausea and vomiting
Diarrhoea
Myalgia
Arthralgia (arthritis is uncommon)
Haemoptysis and pleuritic pain are uncommon

SIGNS

Fever
Respiratory crackles
Tachypnoea
Rash in 25% (may be erythema multiforme)
Tympanic membrane inflammation in 20%
Conjunctivitis
Pharyngitis
Cervical lymphadenopathy

INVESTIGATIONS

FBC
Hb often ↓ (haemolysis)
WCC sometimes ↑ (neutrophilia or normal
  differential)
Platelets occasionally ↓
Reticulocytes ↑ in haemolysis

U + Es
Usually normal

LFTs
Bilirubin sometimes ↑ (unconjugated)

ESR ↑
Cold agglutinins present in 50%
Coombs' test often positive
VDRL occasional false positive

Haptoglobins low or absent in haemolysis

CXR
Shows patchy infiltrates, often lower lobe. Bilateral in 20%. Appearance is unhelpful in distinguishing *Mycoplasma* from other causes of pneumonia.

DIAGNOSIS

Usually by complement fixation test (CFT). Single high titre or fourfold rise in titre is diagnostic. Organism can also be cultured from sputum in specific broth but this is not usually used routinely.

DIFFERENTIAL DIAGNOSIS

Other causes of pneumonia.

COMPLICATIONS

Haemolytic anaemia
Meningitis, myelitis, cranial nerve palsies
Ascending paralysis
Polio like illness
Acute glomerulonephritis
Tubo-ovarian abscess
Myocarditis, pericarditis (<5%)
Pancreatitis
Hepatitis
DIC

Death rate is very low. Illness may be prolonged in patients with hypogammaglobulinaemia. Patients with sickle cell disease may have a severe haemolytic crisis, due to cold agglutinin induced haemolysis, together with the hypoxia resulting from the chest infection leading to severe sickling and further haemolysis.

TREATMENT

Macrolides (erythromycin, clarithromycin,
  azithromycin)
Tetracyclines

QUESTION SPOTTING

Grey case
May present as:

Chest infection plus anaemia

Chest infection plus rashes

Chest infection that does not respond to amoxycillin

Chest infection with multisystem involvement in a patient who is otherwise not particularly unwell.

Data interpretation

May present as:

Haemolytic anaemia

and/or deranged LFTs in the presence of chest signs or symptoms. Note that this combination can occur in any type of pneumonia

Chest infection plus haemolytic anaemia: think of *Mycoplasma* pneumonia

Pneumocystis carinii resembles both fungi and protozoa. Infection is common and usually asymptomatic, but can be life threatening in the immunocompromised host. Cell mediated immunity is required to prevent clinical disease. It is one of the most common diseases to occur in HIV infected patients and is one of the AIDS defining diseases.

It usually remains confined to the lungs where it causes pneumonitis, rarely becoming disseminated. The organism may remain dormant for years and then reactivate when immunosuppression occurs.

SYMPTOMS

Triad of:

Fever
Shortness of breath
Cough – persistent and usually non-productive

Disease may be preceded by upper respiratory tract infection or diarrhoea, and may run a subacute course.

SIGNS

Fever
Tachypnoea
Cyanosis
Crackles in the chest are rare

INVESTIGATIONS

FBC
Hb normal
WBC not useful as may be ↑ or ↓
Platelets normal

U + Es
Normal

LFTs
Normal

ABGs
May be normal at rest, but desaturation occurs on exertion

Chest X-ray
May be the typical appearance of diffuse alveolar shadowing, starting at the hila and spreading from there. The apices and bases are spared until late in the disease. Other recognized features include local infiltrate, nodule, cavity or pneumothorax. The radiograph appearance lags behind the clinical disease and may be normal.

DIAGNOSIS

Cytology is essential for diagnosis. This usually requires bronchoscopy and bronchoalveolar lavage. The cysts are seen with a silver stain as black spheres.

Immunofluorescence and PCR are highly sensitive and specific.

TREATMENT

Oxygen.
HIV testing if no other cause for immunocompromise.
Intravenous high dose co-trimoxazole. Treatment can switch to oral once the patient is responding.
Alternative treatment is pentamidine, but this has a high rate of side effects.
Steroids may have a useful role in reducing mortality in patients with respiratory failure.

Prophylaxis is required following the acute attack as the organism is never eliminated. Oral co-trimoxazole is effective or oral dapsone and pyrimethamine is also useful. Inhaled pentamidine can also be inhaled for prophylaxis.
Primary prevention should be given to HIV infected patients with CD4 count <200/mm^3

PROGNOSIS

100% mortality without treatment
5–15% mortality with treatment

DIFFERENTIAL DIAGNOSIS

CMV
TB

Other bacterial, viral or fungal infection, e.g. Cryptococcus, Histoplasmosis, Aspergillosis.
Pneumonitis secondary to drugs, esp. cytotoxic drugs, e.g. methotrexate.

QUESTION SPOTTING

Grey case

Watch out for PCP in unwell patients with shortness of breath but no respiratory signs and a normal chest X-ray. 'Young man' in a question should make you consider HIV infection, and look for other features suggestive of HIV infection such as weight loss, and candida infection. Normal oxygen saturations at rest do not exclude the diagnosis.

Data interpretation

Unlikely to occur in this section.

ALPHA-1-ANTITRYPSIN DEFICIENCY

α1-Antitrypsin (α1AT) is an inhibitor of neutrophil elastase. One in ten of the population carries a mutation – the M allele produces a normal amount of protein, Z produces 15% and S produces 40% of normal. Homozygotes for the Z mutation occur at a rate of one per 2500 population. Unopposed neutrophil elastase activity leads to accelerated lung damage, especially in smokers, with consequent emphysema. The Z mutation also accumulates in hepatocytes, leading to hepatocyte death and cirrhosis. Heterozygotes for Z produce less severe disease, but may result in cirrhosis.

SYMPTOMS

Progressive SOB, wheeze
Weight loss

Late onset
Jaundice, abdominal swelling
Ankle oedema (cor pulmonale and cirrhosis)

SIGNS

Wheeze, reduced breath sounds
Hyperexpanded chest
Signs of cor pulmonale (late)
Jaundice
Spider naevi
Palmar erythema
Ascites
Encephalopathy (late)

INVESTIGATIONS

FBC
Hb $\uparrow$ in severe lung disease
WCC normal
Platelets usually normal

U + Es
Normal

LFTs
May all be elevated
INR raised in cirrhosis

ECG may reflect cor pulmonale (RVH, p pulmonale)
CXR shows basal emphysematous changes
PFTs show reduced FEV_1/FVC ratio. Reduced TLco

DIAGNOSIS

Liver biopsy shows diastase resistant PAS positive inclusions in hepatocytes, together with evidence of cirrhosis. α1AT mutations are detected by isoelectric focusing on gel electrophoresis.

ASSOCIATIONS

Bronchiectasis
Glomerulonephritis
Panniculitis
Inflammatory bowel disease
Wegener's granulomatosis

TREATMENT

Avoid smoking (accelerates disease)
Avoid excessive alcohol
Avoid pyrexia in infants (high temperatures are thought to encourage deposition of Z protein in the liver, contributing to the infantile hepatitis and liver dysfunction seen in ZZ homozygotes)

PROGNOSIS

10% of infants who are ZZ homozygotes become jaundiced during the first year of life. 10–15% of these develop juvenile cirrhosis; the rest appear to recover at least partially.

50% of adults with ZZ will eventually develop cirrhosis. Hepatocellular carcinoma may develop as a result.

In ZZ disease, emphysema typically becomes apparent at age around 50. In smokers, the onset may be much younger

QUESTION SPOTTING

Grey case
The combination of emphysema and liver dysfunction is usually a pointer to α1AT deficiency. Watch out for emphysema in a young person, especially if they do not smoke.

Data interpretation
May present as obstructive PFTs which are not reversible with salbutamol in a young person.

EXTRINSIC ALLERGIC ALVEOLITIS

A hypersensitivity reaction to inhaled dusts, which may be inorganic but are usually organic. Examples include fungal spores from mouldy hay (farmer's lung), avian proteins (pigeon fancier's lung) and sugar (bagassosis). An acute illness may occur, mediated by a type III hypersensitivity reaction, and a chronic inflammatory disease process also occurs, leading to granuloma formation and lung fibrosis. Many asymptomatic exposures to the antigen may occur before the onset of an acute episode.

ACUTE ILLNESS

Symptoms – onset 2–12 h after exposure
Dry cough
Flu like illness
SOB
Fever
Myalgia
Wheeze is uncommon

Signs
Fever
Bibasal crackles

CHRONIC ILLNESS

Symptoms
Cough
Insidious SOB
Fatigue
Weight loss

Signs
Crackles may be absent
Clubbing is uncommon until late in disease
Signs of right heart failure occur in advanced disease

INVESTIGATIONS

FBC
Hb normal
WCC neutrophilia (in acute illness only)
No eosinophilia
Platelets normal

U + Es
Normal

LFTs
Normal
Calcium normal

Immunoglobulins normal
Serum precipitins (IgG) may be positive

CXR
Shows bibasal alveolar shadowing in acute illness. May be normal.
Reticulonodular shadowing in chronic illness; often in upper and middle zones.
Lymphadenopathy is not a feature

PFTs
Show reduced TLco and FVC in acute and chronic disease. Occasionally, FEV_1 may be disproportionately reduced.

DIAGNOSIS

For acute attacks, diagnosis rests on a typical history, evidence of exposure to an antigen, and whether avoidance of the antigen stops the acute attacks. An inhalational antigen challenge is occasionally necessary; this should reproduce features of an acute attack.

Chronic disease may be more difficult to diagnose; occasionally, lung biopsy is necessary; this shows granulomas, fibrosis and may show bronchiolitis obliterans. High resolution CT may demonstrate fibrosis.

Serum precipitins are not diagnostic of EAA; they merely denote exposure to the relevant antigen. Incidence of exposure to antigens is many times higher than the incidence of clinically overt disease. Absence of the relevant precipitins militates against the diagnosis however.

DIFFERENTIAL DIAGNOSIS

Cryptogenic fibrosing alveolitis
Sarcoidosis
Tuberculosis
Atypical pneumonia
Pneumoconioses
Pulmonary vasculitis
Pulmonary alveolar proteinosis

TREATMENT

Avoidance of the triggering antigen is the mainstay of treatment. Steroids can curtail an acute attack; they may have a role in attenuating chronic disease, but once fibrotic changes occur, the course of the chronic disease tends to be slowly progressive.

PROGNOSIS

Acute attacks usually resolve in 12–48 h, leaving no residual lung damage. Chronic disease may progress to end stage lung fibrosis with cor pulmonale.

QUESTION SPOTTING

Grey case

A person with pets, birds or an interesting looking environmental history or occupation (not just farmers!), who presents with an acute respiratory illness, may have EAA. Note that the presence of precipitins does not necessarily mean that the diagnosis is EAA.

Data interpretation

As above. The presence of a restrictive defect with impaired gas transfer suggests lung fibrosis; the short story may suggest a diagnosis.

OBSTRUCTIVE SLEEP APNOEA

This disorder is due to recurrent collapse of the walls of the pharynx during sleep, causing respiratory obstruction.

The most important cause is obesity but others include hypothyroidism, acromegaly, enlarged tonsils or SVC obstruction. Rarely the condition is familial, and these patients have set back mandibles and maxillas, narrowing their upper airways. Nasal obstruction by adenoids, rhinitis, polyps or nasal deformities may also precipitate the disorder.

SYMPTOMS

Triad of
Hypersomnolence
Heavy snoring
Restless sleep

Other symptoms
Morning headaches secondary to CO_2 retention
Depression
Disorientation
Nocturnal enuresis
Loss of libido
Impotence
Palpitations from tachyarrhythmias

SIGNS

Obesity
Features of causative condition if present

INVESTIGATIONS

FBC
Hb $\uparrow$
WCC normal
Platelets normal

U + Es
Normal

LFTs
Normal

ABGs
pO_2 normal or $\downarrow$
pCO_2 normal or $\uparrow$
pH may be $\uparrow$

Exclude other conditions in differential diagnosis by metabolic testing and throat examination.

DIAGNOSIS

Sleep studies for oxygen saturations and observation. EEG, EMG, ECG, eye movements and air flow may also be measured but are not thought to be essential for the diagnosis. Diagnosis requires more than 15 apnoeas of more than 10 s per hour of sleep.

ECG recording shows cyclical R-R variation.

DIFFERENTIAL DIAGNOSIS

Nocturnal myoclonus – repeated leg movements during sleep that disrupt sleep pattern and produce daytime somnolence.

Narcolepsy – sleep attacks, cataplexy (sudden loss of muscular tone associated with emotion), sleep paralysis and hypnagogic hallucinations.

Idiopathic hypersomnolence.

Laryngeal obstruction from complications of rheumatoid arthritis or Shy-Drager syndrome.

COMPLICATIONS

Cor pulmonale
Hypertension
Polycythemia
Respiratory failure especially if pre-existing respiratory obstruction such as asthma or chronic airway obstruction

TREATMENT

Treatment of underlying cause if acromegaly, myxoedema, enlarged tonsils or SVC obstruction
Weight loss
Avoidance of respiratory depressants, sedatives and muscle relaxants such as alcohol, strong analgesics, and benzodiazepines
Continuous nasal positive airways pressure via a nasal mask at night is effective if tolerated
Tricyclic antidepressants may be effective if only mild
Surgery (uvulo-palato-pharyngoplasty) is advocated by some centres but is not proven to be effective

Tracheostomy is effective but not without its own problems. However it may be life saving as a temporary measure whilst treating the underlying cause of the apnoea.

QUESTION SPOTTING

Grey case

Obstructive sleep apnoea may masquerade in the grey cases as a cause of daytime confusion, loss of concentration or depression. Do not confuse with narcolepsy which has a different clinical pattern.

Data interpretation

If shown nocturnal oxygenation chart, this should be an easy spot diagnosis.

ALLERGIC BRONCHOPULMONARY ASPERGILLOSIS

Aspergillosis is usually caused by the fungus *Aspergillus fumigatus* and rarely causes disease in immunocompetent non-atopic people. However, it may cause a wide array of clinical syndromes depending on the host. The most important of these include allergic bronchopulmonary aspergillosis (ABPA), invasive aspergillosis which may be local or generalized, and aspergillomas. ABPA is caused by the inhalation and trapping of spores in the viscid secretions of atopic and cystic fibrosis patients.

ABPA affects up to 20% of patients with asthma. Men and women are equally affected. Most patients are less than 35 years old at presentation.

SYMPTOMS

Low grade fever
Cough productive of brown mucus plugs
Wheezing
Increasing shortness of breath
Pleuritic chest pain
Haemoptysis

SIGNS

Diffuse wheeze
Prolonged expiratory phase
Crackles are only heard when pulmonary
   infiltrates are present
Finger clubbing may occur if fibrosis

INVESTIGATIONS

FBC
Hb normal
WCC normal or ↑ but eosinophils ↑↑
   (>1.0 × 10⁹/L)
Platelets normal

U + Es
Normal

LFTs
Total protein may be ↑

IgE ↑
ESR ↑
Sputum samples show fungal hyphae on
   microscopy (not a specific test)

Chest X-ray
Transient patchy infiltrates with or without collapse or consolidation. More common in upper lobes. Bronchiectasis of proximal airways may be seen. Fibrosis with honeycombing also occurs later on.

High resolution CT may show bronchiectasis, fibrosis and infiltrates.

Lung function tests show a reversible obstructive defect.

Bronchoscopy and lavage shows positive culture to *Aspergillus fumigatus*, numerous hyphae, mononuclear cells and eosinophils.

DIAGNOSIS

Diagnosis requires a positive skin prick test (beware high false positive rate), increased total IgE with increased IgE and IgG to *Aspergillus* species (serum precipitins). Radiological evidence of APBA with the appropriate clinical features are also required.

DIFFERENTIAL DIAGNOSIS

Churg-Strauss syndrome
Tuberculosis
Sarcoid
Parasitic infestation
Extrinsic allergic alveolitis
Eosinophilic pneumonia
Bacterial infection
Invasive pulmonary aspergillosis

COMPLICATIONS

Bronchiectasis secondary to immune complex
   deposition
Upper lobe fibrosis and honeycomb lung
Cor pulmonale (rare)
Haemoptysis (rare)

TREATMENT

Oral corticosteroids (prednisolone 30–40 mg) for 2 weeks initially and then tapered to control symptoms.

PROGNOSIS

Remission is usual after steroids, but exacerbations are common, and may occur up to 7 years after the acute stage. Progression to steroid dependence (to control asthma or ABPA or both) is not uncommon, and this may eventually lead to pulmonary fibrosis, cor pulmonale and death, though this is rare.

QUESTION SPOTTING

Grey case

The typical patient will be young and will have asthma or cystic fibrosis. The most common scenario will be abnormalities on a chest X-ray in the absence of extra clinical features, or an exacerbation of shortness of breath with other features such as mucus production and fever. Remember to work out eosinophil counts if part of a blood differential is given.

Data interpretation

Less likely to appear in this section.

GASTRIC DISEASE

3

PRIMARY BILIARY CIRRHOSIS

An autoimmune disease of unknown aetiology. PBC is characterized by granulomatous destruction of small intrahepatic bile ducts, leading to slowly progressive cholestasis and eventual cirrhosis. 90% of patients are female, with a peak age of onset of 40–60 years

SYMPTOMS

PBC is often asymptomatic at presentation

Early
Pruritus (usually first symptom)
Tiredness

Late
Jaundice
Haematemesis
Abdominal discomfort
Steatorrhoea

SIGNS

Hepatomegaly
Splenomegaly
Scratch marks
Other signs of chronic liver disease
Xanthelasma
Clubbing
Jaundice, ascites and oedema are all late findings

INVESTIGATIONS

FBC
Usually normal but all counts reduced in
    hypersplenism

U + Es
Usually normal

LFTs
ALP ↑, usually markedly
ALT slightly ↑
Bilirubin ↑ later in disease
Gamma GT ↑
Albumin ↓ in cirrhosis

Cholesterol ↑
INR ↑ in decompensating cirrhosis
IgM often ↑
Immune complexes normal
Serum ACE may be ↑

Antinuclear antibody may be positive, and many other antibodies may be found, including anti-SSA (Ro), anticentromere, antithyroid and antiAChR antibodies.

DIAGNOSIS

Antimitochondrial antibody is positive in 95%. Specificity of the M2 subtype is 98%; this antibody is found at low titre in autoimmune hepatitis.

Liver biopsy shows granulomas, small bile duct destruction, progressing to piecemeal necrosis and cirrhosis.

ASSOCIATIONS

Gallstones
Breast carcinoma

Almost any autoimmune process can be associated:

Sicca syndrome (75%)
Thyroiditis (20%)
Rheumatoid arthritis
SLE
Dermatomyositis
Scleroderma/CREST
Autoimmune thrombocytopenia
Addison's disease
Fibrosing alveolitis
IgA deficiency
Membranous glomerulonephritis
Ulcerative colitis
Transverse myelitis
Renal tubular acidosis
Coeliac disease
Lichen planus
Graves' disease
Myasthenia gravis

DIFFERENTIAL DIAGNOSIS

Chronic viral hepatitis
Primary sclerosing cholangitis
Autoimmune hepatitis
Sarcoidosis
Drug reactions

COMPLICATIONS

Portal hypertension leading to varices
Hepatic encephalopathy
Ascites
Oedema
Renal tubular acidosis
Osteoporosis
Hypercholesterolaemia
Osteomalacia (longstanding severe disease only)

TREATMENT

Cholestyramine relieves pruritus.
    Liver transplantation: 85–90% survival at
1 year. Recurrence is rare. Consider when
bilirubin >100 μmol/L.
    Ursodeoxycholic acid is somewhat
controversial, but may prolong the interval
before death or liver transplant.
    Methotrexate may also be of value, but
cyclosporin, colchicine and steroids do not
appear to improve prognosis, although they may
improve symptoms.

PROGNOSIS

Asymptomatic patients: 10–16 year median
    survival
Symptomatic patients: 7 year median survival

QUESTION SPOTTING

Grey case

PBC must be on the differential of any grey case
involving a woman with liver disease. Other
features to look for are:

Pruritus in a middle aged woman
ALP and hepatomegaly without a very high
    bilirubin

Liver disease with a number of other
autoimmune conditions, especially
hypothyroidism, dry eyes or scleroderma.

Data interpretation

Once again, the clue is usually a raised ALP
without a large rise in bilirubin. Look for a raised
cholesterol as supporting evidence, perhaps with
a raised IgM.
    An alternative scenario is the addition of
urinary biochemistry depicting renal tubular
acidosis; haemochromatosis and Wilson's
disease are two other causes of RTA with liver
involvement.

AUTOIMMUNE HEPATITIS

An autoimmune disease of unknown aetiology. It may have either a chronic or acute, fulminant course. Histology shows piecemeal necrosis in zone one of the hepatic parenchyma, with a lymphocytic infiltrate.

SYMPTOMS

Tiredness
Anorexia
Nausea
Jaundice, RUQ tenderness and abdominal
    distension may occur in acute illness

SIGNS

Palmar erythema
Spider naevi
Hepatomegaly
Splenomegaly
Moon face, abdominal striae and central obesity
    may be evident even without steroid treatment

INVESTIGATIONS

FBC
Hb ↓
MCV normal
WCC usually normal – ↓ in hypersplenism
Platelets usually normal – ↓ in hypersplenism

U + Es
Normal

LFTs
Bilirubin ↑ in 25–50% at presentation
ALT ↑ 2–20 times normal
ALP slightly ↑
Albumin low

INR ↑ in advanced disease
ESR ↑

IgG ↑
IgA, IgM usually normal

Antibodies
ANA positive in 40–70%
Anti-smooth muscle antibodies positive in 60%
Anti-LKM-1 antibodies may also be positive
Anti-mitochondrial antibodies occasionally
    positive at low titre

DIAGNOSIS

Liver biopsy shows lymphocyte infiltration, piecemeal necrosis, and fibrosis as the disease progresses. The biliary tree is relatively spared.

Presence of features of hepatitis, anti-smooth muscle antibodies and typical histology usually clinch the diagnosis.

ASSOCIATIONS

Other autoimmune conditions are present in 60%
    of cases of autoimmune hepatitis
Sicca syndrome (35%)
Renal tubular acidosis (24%)
Peripheral neuropathy (10%)
Hashimoto's thyroiditis (7%)
Ulcerative colitis (4%)
Rheumatoid arthritis (2%)
Thrombocytopenia/haemolytic anaemia
Mixed connective tissue disease
Diabetes mellitus
Diabetes insipidus
Graves' disease
Pulmonary fibrosis
Coeliac disease
Myasthenia gravis
Polymyositis
Glomerulonephritis

DIFFERENTIAL DIAGNOSIS

Acute disease
Hepatitis A, B, C, E infection
EBV/CMV hepatitis
Wilson's disease
Drug toxicity

Chronic disease
Chronic hepatitis B/C
Primary biliary cirrhosis (PBC)
Primary sclerosing cholangitis
Wilson's disease
α1-Antitrypsin deficiency
Alcohol abuse

Note that overlap syndromes, especially with PBC, are recognized.

COMPLICATIONS

Cirrhosis with other features of liver failure.
Varices with associated bleeding may occur
Hepatocellular carcinoma
Hypersplenism
Hepatic encephalopathy may complicate acute or
end stage disease

TREATMENT

Steroids, with azathioprine as a steroid sparing
agent once in remission.
Liver transplantation is successful for end stage
disease.

PROGNOSIS

>95% 10 year survival if no cirrhosis present
65% 10 year survival if cirrhosis present

QUESTION SPOTTING

Grey case

Acute or chronic liver disease, especially in a
young woman, should lead to consideration of
autoimmune hepatitis.
Pointers to the diagnosis are:

Negative viral serology
Markedly raised ALT/AST
High immunoglobulin levels (or large difference
between total protein and albumin)
Presence of anti-smooth muscle antibodies
No history of drugs or alcohol

Data interpretation

The above points apply.

HEREDITARY HAEMOCHROMATOSIS

Hereditary condition leading to inappropriately high absorption of iron by the gut mucosa with increased transfer of iron to plasma. This leads to excessive total body iron and deposition of iron in cells of the liver, heart, pancreas, joints, skin, gonads and other endocrine organs. This in turn causes tissue damage, fibrosis and functional failure. The deposition in parenchymal cells of the liver contrasts with normal individuals who tend to deposit iron in the bone marrow. Liver damage is fibrotic. Hepatitis suggests viral infection or alcohol abuse.

The candidate gene HFE has recently been found and is located on chromosome 6p21, closely linked with HLA A3. There is a lesser linkage with HLA B14. 80–90% of patients have a single mutation at site 282. Heterozygotes have increased iron absorption without the disease. (25% have abnormal iron studies.)

Women are protected by menstruation and so present clinically later than men.

SYMPTOMS

Often asymptomatic
Weakness
Lethargy
Abdominal pain
Arthralgia
Loss of libido and impotence
Symptoms of cardiac failure
Symptoms of diabetes such as thirst and polyuria

SIGNS

Hepatomegaly
Splenomegaly
Loss of body hair
Gynaecomastia
Testicular atrophy
Skin pigmentation – 'bronze'
Arthritis
Signs of diabetes mellitus

INVESTIGATIONS

FBC
Normal

U + Es
Normal

Glucose normal or ↑

LFTs
AST ↑
ALP ↑
Bilirubin ↑
Albumin normal

Iron↑
Ferritin ↑
TIBC ↓
Fasting transferrin saturation ↑
(iron ÷ TIBC × 100%)

Testosterone ↓

Urine iron excretion ↑ after desferrioxamine

Joint X-rays show cartilage calcification

Dual energy CT scan (which requires modifications to the CT scanner for the test) has high correlation for iron overload, but is less sensitive for lower levels.

Magnetic susceptibility is available in some units (SQUID – super conducting quantum interference device)

DIAGNOSIS

Liver biopsy with iron staining and biochemical measurement of hepatic iron concentration (HIC)
Hepatic iron index (HII) (HIC ÷ patient age) (If >1.9 highly suggestive of hereditary haemochromatosis but false negative rate of 10%)

DIFFERENTIAL DIAGNOSIS

Chronic liver disease, e.g. alcoholic cirrhosis, chronic viral hepatitis, post porto-caval shunt
Parenteral iron overdose (intravenous iron, transfusions, haemodialysis)
Ineffective erythropoiesis, e.g. thalassaemia major, sideroblastic anaemia treated by blood transfusion
Porphyria cutanea tarda
Congenital atransferrinaemia
Neonatal iron overload
African iron overload (inherited, non-HLA linked)

COMPLICATIONS

Cirrhosis of the liver – later in women
Cardiac – restrictive cardiomyopathy,
    arrhythmias, and cardiac failure
Diabetes mellitus
Hepatocellular carcinoma ($200 \times$ risk)
Rarely cholangiocarcinoma
Chondrocalcinosis and degenerative joint disease
Infertility in men
Patients are also at greater risk of certain
    infections, especially, hepatitis B and C,
    listeria and yersinia.

TREATMENT

Weekly phlebotomy of 500 ml of blood until
erythrocytosis is iron dependent (i.e.
haemoglobin or haematocrit do not recover by
the next phlebotomy). Monitor the transferrin
saturation and ferritin. Continue phlebotomy
until transferrin saturation is <50% or ferritin
<50 ng/ml. Then bleed 500 ml blood every
2–3 months.

Avoid alcohol and vitamin C which can
increase iron absorption.

Liver transplant may be considered but results
are poor with only 50–60% survival rates.

PROGNOSIS

Normal prognosis if no cirrhosis and compliant
with treatment.

QUESTION SPOTTING

Grey case

The typical patient will be a male in his 40s who
presents with cirrhotic liver disease, who will
have incidental findings of diabetes. These two
findings should immediately alert you to the
possibility of haemochromatosis. Other findings
such as cardiac failure, arthralgia, skin
pigmentation, gonadal failure or
chondrocalcinosis will strengthen suspicion. The
diagnosis will only definitively be made on liver
biopsy.

Data interpretation

May be asked to interpret the iron profile results
and suggest a diagnosis of haemochromatosis.

WILSON'S DISEASE (HEPATOLENTICULAR DEGENERATION)

An autosomal recessive disease caused by a posttranslational defect in caeruloplasmin production. This leads to failure of hepatocyte excretion of copper into the bile. Copper accumulates in the liver and when saturated, in other organs, notably the brain, cornea and lens, kidney, red blood cells, bones, and skin.

Onset is usually between 6 and 40 years of age and the clinical picture can be very variable.

SIGNS

Hepatic
Hepatitis
Cirrhosis
Portal hypertension with splenomegaly, varices and ascites
Pigment gallstones from haemolysis.
Hepatocellular carcinoma – rare in contrast to haemochromatosis

Central nervous system
Tremor
Dysarthria
Drooling
Chorea
Dystonic spasms or posturing
Akinesia
Rigidity
Seizures
Personality change and behaviour disturbance
Dementia – late
Hearing, vision and sensation are not usually affected
Reflexes are usually normal as are the plantar responses

Ocular
Kayser-Fleischer rings
Sunflower cataracts

Renal
Renal tubular acidosis (usually proximal) with osteomalacia/rickets

Haematological
Haemolytic anaemia (10%). This is typically non-spherocytic and Coomb's negative.

Skin
Copper deposition leads to bluish tinging, and blue lunulae in the nailbeds.

Other features
Osteoarthritis of the spine (Scheuermann's disease)
Polyarthritis
Hypermobile joints
Chondromalacia patellae

INVESTIGATIONS

FBC
Normal

U + Es
Normal

LFTs
Bilirubin $\uparrow$
AST $\uparrow$
ALP $\uparrow$
Albumin $\downarrow$
Clotting prolonged if severe liver disease
Bicarb $\downarrow$ if RTA
Caeruloplasmin $\downarrow$
Total copper $\downarrow$ (or normal)
Free copper $\uparrow\uparrow$

Urinalysis
Glucose +
Protein +
Amino acids +
$\uparrow$ urinary 24 h copper (may be raised in other chronic liver disease and in proteinuria)

CT/MRI brain scans show cerebral atrophy and degeneration of basal ganglia.

DIAGNOSIS

Liver biopsy shows $\uparrow\uparrow$ copper levels (>250 mcg/g dry weight)

TREATMENT

Penicillamine for life.
Trientine may be used if penicillamine intolerant.

Some clinicians advise potassium sulphide or zinc as additional therapy, as they reduce copper absorption in the gut.

A low copper diet is also advised.

Some worsening in symptoms may be seen early on in treatment and response is rare before 6–12 months. Treatment may be reduced once copper levels are normalized but should be continued for life. Even apparently severe liver and central nervous disease are potentially reversible.

Liver transplant is useful in young patients with severe disease, especially as it corrects the metabolic defect, so that treatment may be stopped.

Relatives of patients with Wilson's disease should be screened.

PROGNOSIS

Death occurs in 5–14 years without treatment.

QUESTION SPOTTING

Grey case

A young patient who has odd neurological symptoms should raise the suspicion of Wilson's disease and this diagnosis should also be considered if liver failure occurs in a young patient where there is no obvious cause.

Data interpretation

May present as a cause of renal tubular acidosis, or hepatitis. Liver disease plus haemolysis should also raise the suspicion of Wilson's disease.

Chronic inflammatory disease invariably affecting the rectum which can spread in a confluent manner to involve the whole colon (pancolitis). Mucosa can return to normal when the inflammation subsides but there is usually some residual glandular distortion.

The cause of ulcerative colitis (and Crohn's disease) is not known, and it is possible that the two diseases represent manifestations of the same disease but different environmental factors determine which disease phenotype occurs. Ulcerative colitis for instance is less likely in smokers, unlike Crohn's disease. However the pathogens implicated in Crohn's disease (mycobacterium and viruses) have not been found in ulcerative colitis. Likewise xANCA (antigen is lactoferrin) is raised in ulcerative colitis but not in Crohn's disease.

SYMPTOMS

Bloody diarrhoea with mucus
Urgency of defecation and tenesmus
Lower abdominal pain
Weight loss
Fever
Malaise
Nausea
Anorexia
Arthritis

SIGNS

May be none
Anaemia
Tachycardia
Fever
Mouth ulcers
Abdominal tenderness
Finger clubbing – rare

INVESTIGATIONS

FBC
Hb ↓ (MCV normal or ↓ if chronic blood loss)
WBC ↑
Platelets normal or ↑

U + Es
Normal

LFTs
Albumin ↓
LFTs abnormal

Differential diagnosis of abnormal LFTs in inflammatory bowel disease
Acute colitis: acute phase response and fatty change
Pericholangitis: mostly benign. Usually in pancolitis and resolves with colectomy
Viral hepatitis: may be transfusion related
Gallstones
Autoimmune cholangiopathy: similar to autoimmune chronic active hepatitis and responds to steroids
Primary sclerosing cholangitis (70% of patients with PSC have UC)
Drug induced
Hepatic granulomas
Liver abscess
Amyloid
ESR and CRP ↑

Stool analysis
Negative for pathogens
Positive for blood

X-rays
AXR
May show colonic dilatation
Sacroiliitis
Ankylosing spondylitis

DIAGNOSIS

Barium
Double contrast study will show abnormal mucosal pattern and ulceration if present. Plain abdominal radiography should precede barium study to exclude toxic dilatation.

Rectal biopsy
Mucosa shows erythema and reduced vascular pattern. Ulcers tend to occur late. Pseudopolyps and mucosal bridging may occur.

DIFFERENTIAL DIAGNOSIS

See Crohn's disease

COMPLICATIONS

Carcinoma 5–10% after 20 years of disease. May be multifocal and often mucinous in type
Abscess formation
Acute toxic bowel rare but commoner than Crohn's
Perforation rare but commoner than Crohn's
Haemorrhage rare but commoner than Crohn's
Fistulae (external, rectovaginal) – very rare unlike Crohn's
Stricture formation – very rare unlike Crohn's

TREATMENT

General medical measures: fluid and electrolyte replacement, blood transfusion as required.

Oral steroids and topical steroids via rectal enemas (only in the acute attack)
Oral aminosalicylate (effective in acute attack and also to maintain remission)

Topical mesalazine enemas if refractory to oral aminosalicylate and topical steroids.

Azathioprine or 6-mercaptopurine are effective steroid sparing agents in maintaining remission in those patients not controlled by aminosalicylates. Cyclosporin is also used to control severe active inflammation not responding to other measures.

Metronidazole has no proven use in ulcerative colitis, and elemental feeding does not reduce disease activity in ulcerative colitis. Cf. Crohn's disease.

Surgery
Absolute indications
Uncontrolled haemorrhage
Perforation
Carcinoma

Relative indications
Severe colitis ± toxic megacolon not responding to maximal medical therapy
Severe intractable symptoms
Intolerable side effects from disease modifying medications

Intolerable extracolonic manifestations, e.g. pyoderma gangrenosum, haemolytic anaemia or arthritis but note the course of primary sclerosing cholangitis is independent of disease activity and colectomy.
Operation may either be a proctocolectomy with ileostomy or total colectomy with ileoanal anastomosis and pouch formation.

QUESTION SPOTTING

Grey case
Either ulcerative colitis or Crohn's disease may be presented and differentiation may be made by clues in the history or the investigation results and by the extraenteric manifestations. Particularly watch for sclerosing cholangitis in UC and gallstones/oxalate renal stones in Crohn's. Either may give a history of arthritis, eye problems or a rash which may be confused with one of the connective tissue disorders.

Data interpretation
Likely to ask about the causes of abnormal liver tests in a patient with inflammatory bowel disease.

CROHN'S DISEASE

Chronic inflammatory disease affecting any part of the gut with special predisposition for the terminal ileum, colon and anorectum.

The cause of Crohn's disease is still not known. A single aetiological factor has not been found and most now believe that the disease is due to poorly regulated immune and inflammatory processes within the gut wall. The initial response is likely to be caused by a bacterial stimulus, but genetically susceptible individuals then suffer from an overexpression of both local immune reactions, and systemic inflammatory cell infiltrate. These continue, unchecked by the normal counter-inflammatory mechanisms.

A possible association is with a low-residue, high refined sugar diet, and a clear link with smoking has been established.

Genetic studies have demonstrated that at least three genes give rise to increased susceptibility to inflammatory bowel disease, and family members with predisposing genotype are as likely to get Crohn's disease as ulcerative colitis. However, the phenotype may be determined by environmental factors, especially smoking.

SYMPTOMS

Diarrhoea
Abdominal pain
Weight loss
Fever
Rectal bleeding especially in colonic disease
Perianal disease
Obstructive symptoms of colic and vomiting especially in ileal disease.
Tiredness and shortness of breath if anaemic
Bone pain secondary to osteomalacia if malabsorption of vitamin D
Excessive bleeding if malabsorption of vitamin K

SIGNS

May be normal
Anaemia
Mouth ulcers
Glossitis
Clubbing of nails
Abdominal tenderness
Palpable abdominal mass, particularly right iliac fossa
Anal fissures, fistulae and skin tags

INVESTIGATIONS

FBC

Hb $\downarrow$ (mixed deficiencies can cause MCV $\uparrow$ or $\downarrow$)
WCC $\uparrow$ (neutrophilia)
Platelets $\uparrow$
B_{12} and folate may be low

U + Es

Na normal
K $\downarrow$ due to diarrhoea
Urea and creatinine normal

LFTs

Bilirubin, AST and ALP $\uparrow$ (especially a mild $\uparrow$ in AST and ALP) (see also UC)
Albumin $\downarrow$ in active disease (due to negative acute phase reaction and protein losing enteropathy)
Calcium $\downarrow$ in severe small bowel disease

Mg^{2+}, Zn^{2+} and selenium may be $\downarrow$
Ferritin is best marker of iron stores but may be $\uparrow$ in acute phase

X-rays

AXR

Intestinal obstruction
Inflammatory mass in right iliac fossa
Mucosal oedema
Ulceration may be seen in acute active Crohn's
Sacroiliitis or ankylosing spondylitis

Sinography

External fistulae

DIAGNOSIS

Barium meal with follow through or infusion (see Fig. 4)
Thickened valvulae coniventes
Small aphthous ulcers
'Rose thorn' ulcers
Cobblestoning
Fissures
Wall thickening

Large bowel should be demonstrated with double contrast barium which typically shows rectal sparing (beware treatment with steroid suppositories) – see example of barium enema in Crohn's disease (Fig. 5).

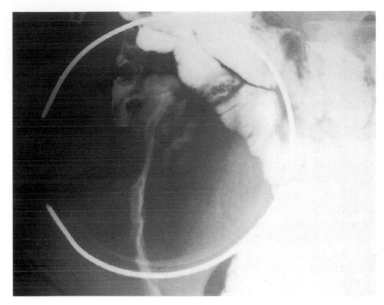

Fig. 4. Crohn's disease. The first X-ray is a barium follow through. The round marker is a compression disc which pushes bowel away from the area of interest. This film shows collapsed severe Crohn's disease of the terminal ileum with the classical string sign. There are multiple 'rose thorn' ulcers, and ulcerated pits. This film also demonstrates area of normal bowel between areas of disease, so called skip lesions. This is typical of Crohn's disease.

Ultrasound useful in demonstrating inflammatory RIF mass and bowel oedema.

Sigmoidoscopy and colonoscopy
Rectal and ileal biopsies.

In the early stages, aphthous ulcers have normal mucosa around them (unlike ulcerative colitis which shows erythema and reduced vascular pattern) and later cobblestoning, fissuring ulcers and oedema are seen. Ulcers tend to be linear and become confluent (ulcerative colitis typically shows inflamed diffuse granular friable dark red mucosa and ulcers only occur in severe disease. Pseudopolyps and mucosal bridges occur in both).

DIFFERENTIAL DIAGNOSIS

Ulcerative colitis
Infective colitis including TB, *Shigella*,
    Campylobacter, *E. coli*, amoebiasis,
    pseudomembranous colitis
Vasculitis including SLE and PAN
Ischaemic colitis
Colonic carcinoma
Collagenous and lymphocytic colitis
Irritable bowel syndrome
Solitary rectal ulcer syndrome
Radiation colitis
Neutropaenic colitis
Diverticulitis
Eosinophilic gastroenteritis
Small bowel lymphoma
Alpha chain disease
Amyloid
Behçet's disease

COMPLICATIONS

Acute toxic bowel, perforation, haemorrhage
    (rare)
Strictures of small or large bowel
Fistulae (enterocolic, gastrocolic, or from bowel
    to bladder or vagina. Can cause pneumaturia
    or faeces in either urine or vaginal discharge)
Involvement of ureters (right > left) may cause
    sterile pyuria, urinary tract infection, or
    ureteric stricture

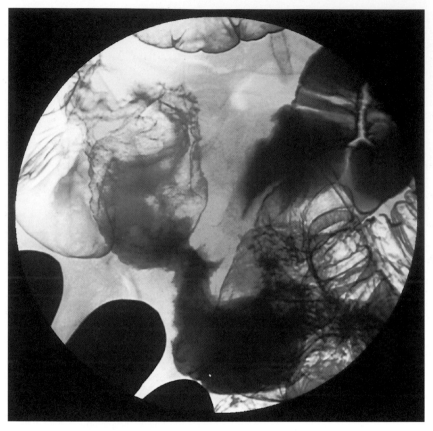

Fig. 5.   Crohn's disease. The second film shows a double contrast barium study. There are more typical 'rose thorn' ulcers. The barium refluxes back into the ileum, which is also abnormal.

Carcinoma (3–5%) in colonic disease. Small bowel carcinoma has also been documented although this is rare

TREATMENT

Stop smoking (will significantly reduce relapse rate)

Diet

Elemental diet is as effective as steroids in acute disease. However it is poorly tolerated, and polymeric diet may have a better compliance. TPN is used if preoperative or severely ill.

Low fibre is used if strictures are present
Low fat is used in steatorrhoea
Vitamin supplements if deficient

Drugs

Steroids in active disease
5-aminosalicylic acid – not very effective except at high doses in active disease
Azathioprine or 6-mercaptopurine for at least 2 years to be effective
Methotrexate is effective but has high incidence of side effects
Metronidazole is proven to be effective in colonic disease but should be given for <3 months due to risk of neuropathy
Broad spectrum antibiotics for small bowel overgrowth
Rectal hydrocortisone enemas

Surgery

70–80% require an operation
Minimal resection margins are recommended

Bypass operations and pouch surgery are
contraindicated

Fistulae should be determined anatomically with
sinograms and only excised after antibiotic
treatment, control of active disease, and
nutrition correction

Colostomy may be useful to defunction bowel
for 12–18 months

Indications

Failure of medical management
Strictures causing obstruction
Fistulae
Abscess or perforation

Extraenteric manifestations and frequencies in Crohn's and ulcerative colitis

Hepatobiliary	Crohn's	UC
Chronic active hepatitis	2–3%	rare
Cirrhosis	5%	20%
Fatty liver	6%	common
Pericholangitis	20%	25%
Primary sclerosing cholangitis	very rare	5–12%
Cholelithiasis	30%	5%
		(normal incidence in population)

Renal		
Oxalate stones		not seen
Ureteric obstruction		not seen
Rheumatological		
Enteropathic arthritis	6–12%	10%
Ankylosing spondylitis	2–6%	2–6%
Sacroiliitis	15–18%	15–18%
Osteoporosis		
Ocular	3–10%	3–10%
Uveitis or iritis		
Episcleritis		
Conjunctivitis		
Dermatological		
Erythema nodosum	5–10%	2%
Pyoderma gangrenosum	0.5%	3%
Aphthous ulceration	20%	seen
Perianal skin tags		rare
Nutrition deficiency diseases		
Other		
Psoas abscess		
Amyloidosis		

QUESTION SPOTTING

See under ulcerative colitis.

BUDD-CHIARI SYNDROME

Obstruction of the larger hepatic veins. This may occur acutely or in a more chronic form.

CAUSES

Unknown in 30%
Thrombosis due to hypercoagulable state –
  polycythemia vera, paroxysmal nocturnal
  haemoglobinuria, and antithrombin III, protein
  C or protein S deficiencies, pregnancy, or oral
  contraceptive pill use.
Malignancy – particularly hepatic, renal and
  adrenal carcinomas.
Congenital venous web – rare outside Japan.
Hepatic infection, e.g. hydatid cysts
Radiotherapy
Trauma

SYMPTOMS

Nausea and vomiting – acute
Upper abdominal pain – acute

SIGNS

Tender hepatomegaly
Ascites
Jaundice – chronic
Splenomegaly – chronic
Peripheral oedema only occurs if inferior vena
  cava involved
Hepatojugular reflex usually absent

INVESTIGATIONS

FBC
Normal

U + Es
Normal

LFTs
Variable
AST ↑
ALP ↑
Bilirubin ↑
Albumin ↓
Ca normal
Clotting may be abnormal

Ascites
Protein >25 g/L initially but falls in chronic phase

DIAGNOSIS

Liver ultrasound
Abdominal CT
MRI
Tc liver scintigram

All can be used to show hepatic vein occlusion and, in the long term, enlargement of the caudate lobe (which has different venous drainage from the rest of the liver). Compression of the inferior vena cava may be present. Pulsed Doppler sonography also shows abnormalities.
  Liver biopsy shows centrilobular congestion with fibrosis.

DIFFERENTIAL DIAGNOSIS

Cirrhosis from other causes
Veno-occlusive disease – rare disease caused by
  widespread non-thrombotic obliteration of the
  central hepatic veins. Pyrrolizidine alkaloids
  (from the plants used to make tea), cytotoxic
  drugs and hepatic irradiation are the most
  common causes. Clinically very similar to
  Budd–Chiari syndrome.
Right-sided cardiac failure
Constrictive pericarditis
Inferior vena cava obstruction

TREATMENT

Treat the underlying cause if identified.
  Ascites should be treated with diuretics, sodium and water restriction, and paracentesis. The ascites may prove difficult to treat, and portal venous shunting by transjugular intrahepatic portasystemic stent shunting (TIPSS) or peritoneal-systemic shunting (the LeVeen procedure).
  Side to side porto-caval or splenorenal anastomosis may be useful to decompress the liver.
  Surgery for congenital webs.
  Rarely thrombolytics such as streptokinase may be tried with subsequent anticoagulation.
  Liver transplantation is becoming more common.

PROGNOSIS

Generally poor. 30–60% die within one year. Survivors may develop cirrhosis.

QUESTION SPOTTING

Grey case

May present with the picture of cirrhosis, but with no obvious underlying cause except that the patient may have some reason for a hypercoagulable state. Also consider if a picture of acute hepatitis occurs with ascites.

Data interpretation

Consider Budd-Chiari if abnormal liver function tests and a liver biopsy which shows centrilobular congestion with or without fibrosis.

COELIAC DISEASE

An autoimmune disease with hypersensitivity to the gliadin fraction of gluten and related products in wheat, rye and barley, characterized by destruction of the normal small bowel mucosal architecture.

Mucosal destruction of the proximal bowel leads to malabsorption of fat, protein and carbohydrate, along with low vitamin A, D, E and K levels, low iron, folate and in severe cases, low B_{12} levels.

There is high prevalence in Ireland and in Punjabi immigrants. There is often a family history.

SYMPTOMS

Many cases are asymptomatic, with anaemia or other disturbances picked up on routine screening tests

Abdominal bloating and discomfort
Diarrhoea and steatorrhoea
Weight loss
Weakness
Anaemic symptoms (tiredness, SOB)
Bone pain
Paraesthesia and tetany if hypocalcaemia
Bruising (from vitamin K coagulopathy)

SIGNS

Anaemia particularly in pregnancy
Proximal muscle weakness (vitamin D malabsorption)
Mouth ulcers and stomatitis
Clubbing (rare)

INVESTIGATIONS

FBC
Hb ↓
WCC and platelets ↓ (folate/B_{12} deficiency)
MCV ↓ if Fe deficient, ↑ if folate/B_{12} deficient.
May be normal if mixed deficiency or mild disease

U + Es
Usually normal
K ↓ in diarrhoea

LFTs
Bilirubin normal
ALP may be ↑ in osteomalacia, or from liver/bowel source
Calcium ↓ or low normal
Albumin often ↓

Fe often ↓
TIBC often ↑
Red cell folate usually ↓
B_{12} may be ↓
Phosphate ↓
IgA often raised, with low IgM levels
INR may be elevated (vitamin K malabsorption)

Blood film
Diamorphic picture if mixed iron deficiency – microcytes, macrocytes, hypersegmented neutrophils.

Features of hyposplenism – target cells, Howell-Jolly bodies, etc.

Barium studies show dilated bowel, smooth outline with prominent (oedematous) valvulae coniventes.

DIAGNOSIS

a) Duodenal biopsy via endoscopy. Histology shows atrophy of villi with crypt hypertrophy. Plasma cells and lymphocytes are seen invading the lamina propria.
b) Anti-gliadin and anti-endomysial antibodies – 90% sensitivity. May be negative in individuals with IgA deficiency (10% of coeliacs).
c) Symptoms improve on a gluten free diet.

ASSOCIATIONS

Dermatitis herpetiformis (gluten sensitive rash)
IDDM
Thyroid disease
Addison's disease
Fibrosing alveolitis
SLE
Polyarteritis
Inflammatory bowel disease
Temporal lobe epilepsy
10% also have IgA deficiency (compared with 0.5% of the general population)

DIFFERENTIAL DIAGNOSIS

Other causes of malabsorption, including:

Crohn's disease
Giardia infection
Post-infectious malabsorption
Whipple's disease
Radiation enteritis
Bacterial overgrowth
Amyloidosis
Lymphoma
Common variable immunodeficiency
Cow's milk intolerance

COMPLICATIONS

Osteoporosis
Osteomalacia
Splenic atrophy
GI lymphoma
Ulcerative jejunoileitis
Oesophageal carcinoma
Pharyngeal carcinoma

TREATMENT

Gluten free diet. Vitamin supplementation may be necessary for 3 to 4 months until the mucosa regenerates. Corticosteroids may be given acutely for severe disease.

QUESTION SPOTTING

Grey case
Present as a generalized malabsorption:

Low folate and iron
Vitamin D deficiency
Steatorrhoea
Weight loss

Often, the difficulty is to distinguish between coeliac disease and the other causes of malabsorption listed above. Look out for:

Recurrent anaemia
A long history, perhaps of poor growth in childhood
No prior history of GI infection
Villous atrophy on small bowel biopsy
Lack of strictures or small bowel surgery
Presence of a rash (dermatitis herpetiformis)
Family history
At risk groups

Data interpretation
Less common, but consider if you see iron, folate, vitamin D deficiency along with raised faecal fats and poor xylose absorption. Again, without further investigations, it is difficult to distinguish coeliac disease from other causes of small bowel malabsorption.

WHIPPLE'S DISEASE

A systemic infection by *Tropheryma whippleii*, a bacterium related to the Actinomycetes. Infection occurs predominantly in males, between the ages of 30 and 70. 98% of cases are in Caucasians, with a predilection for HLA B27 positive individuals. Manual workers with heavy exposure to soil (e.g. builders) are at increased risk.

SYMPTOMS

Abdominal pain
Weight loss (90%)
Arthralgia (80%)
Steatorrhoea/diarrhoea (75%)
Fever (50%)
Confusion, dementia (40%)
Visual impairment (40%)
Lethargy (40%)
Gait disturbance (40%)
Chest pain
SOB

SIGNS

Lymphadenopathy (50%)
Hyperpigmentation (50%)
Cachexia
Arthritis (often a migratory polyarthritis)
Ataxia
Ophthalmoplegia
Abdominal distension
Cardiac murmurs
Bruising
Hypotension (late feature)
Splenomegaly, hepatomegaly (uncommon)

INVESTIGATIONS

FBC
Hb often ↓
MCV normal or ↓
WCC may be ↑
Platelets usually normal

U + Es
Usually normal

LFTs
Bilirubin usually normal

ALT mildly ↑
ALP mildly ↑
Albumin usually ↓
Calcium occasionally ↓ (vitamin D malabsorption)

ESR ↑
CRP ↑
INR may be ↑ (vitamin K malabsorption)
Immunoglobulins may be ↓, normal or elevated
Fe usually low ↓
TIBC ↑
Ferritin ↑
Folate sometimes ↓
B12 may be ↓
Serum ACE may be elevated

Stool fat often elevated (90%)

Urinalysis shows protein and/or microscopic haematuria

CSF shows elevated protein, lymphocytosis

CXR may show mediastinal involvement
Joint XRs show osteoporosis. Arthritis is usually not destructive
Small bowel follow through shows oedematous small bowel, especially jejunum.
U/S abdomen/CT abdomen show thickened small bowel and retroperitoneal lymphadenopathy

DIAGNOSIS

Small bowel biopsy (e.g. distal duodenum) shows diastase resistant PAS positive macrophages. Bacilli visible in the lamina propria (non-acid fast). Distorted villous architecture. Granulomas are usually seen.
Diagnosis can be confirmed by PCR of biopsy or CSF.

DIFFERENTIAL DIAGNOSIS

Coeliac disease and other causes of malabsorption
Malignancy, e.g. lymphoma, lung carcinoma
Sarcoidosis
AIDS
MAI complex bowel infection

Crohn's disease
Addison's disease

COMPLICATIONS

Eye involvement: keratitis, uveitis, retinitis
Cardiac involvement: endocarditis, myocarditis,
    pericarditis
Malabsorption: fat, amino acids, vitamins A, D,
    K, B_{12}, folate
Neurological involvement: dementia, ataxia,
    hemiparesis, personality change,
    ophthalmoplegia
IgA nephropathy, glomerulonephritis and
    interstitial nephritis may occur
Amyloidosis (AA) is a sequel of longstanding
    disease

TREATMENT

Prolonged course of antibiotics which can cross
the blood-brain barrier, e.g. 2 weeks of IV
benzylpenicillin plus streptomycin, followed by
1–2 years of oral co-trimoxazole. Resistant or
relapsing cases may respond to antibiotics plus
interferon gamma.

PROGNOSIS

Untreated, the disease is usually fatal.
    Treated, most patients recover fully, though
this may take 1–2 years. Relapse, especially of
CNS disease, occurs and is still occasionally
fatal.

QUESTION SPOTTING

Grey case
Clues to Whipple's are:

Malabsorption plus:
    Arthritis
    Neurological symptoms
    Cardiac problems, e.g. endocarditis
    Middle aged male patient

Data interpretation
Unlikely to crop up in this section.

CHRONIC PANCREATITIS

Unlike acute pancreatitis, the chronic inflammation in this disease leads to progressive and irreversible structural damage with permanent impairment of endocrine and exocrine function. The pancreatic acini are destroyed by the chronic fibrotic process. The pancreatic ducts become dilated and irregular, and protein plugs and calcification may appear. Clinical evidence of pancreatic exocrine insufficiency occurs after loss of >90% of function. Deficiencies of fat soluble vitamins (A, D, E and K) are possible, but very rare cf. malabsorption such as coeliac disease. Pancreatic endocrine insufficiency occurs and although glucose intolerance is common, overt diabetes mellitus occurs very late in the disease. Patients are also glucagon deficient (unlike idiopathic insulin dependent diabetes), and so are at more risk of treatment related hypoglycaemia.

CAUSES

Alcohol (70–80%)
Idiopathic (10–20%) – bimodal distribution, men=women, some patients found to have a mutation in the cystic fibrosis gene without having cystic fibrosis.
Patients with overt cystic fibrosis
Other (5–10%) include:
Hyperlipidaemia – especially hypertriglyceridaemia
Hereditary – rare, autosomal dominant
Tropical – rare in UK, but common in parts of Africa and Asia. Affects children who are malnourished and cassava fruit has been implicated. Abdominal pain is less frequent.
Obstructive
Chronic hypercalcaemia, e.g. hyperparathyroidism – occurs in 10–15% of these patients if untreated.
Haemochromatosis
Trauma
Post surgical
Pancreas divisum – failure of fusion of the two embryonic parts to the pancreas. Only a small proportion progress to chronic pancreatitis.
Gastrinoma
Alpha-1-antitrypsin deficiency
Deficiencies of amylase, lipase, trypsinogen or enterokinase

SYMPTOMS

Abdominal pain – highly variable pattern
Anorexia
Weight loss – often due to fear of eating
Nausea and vomiting
Mild fever common
Steatorrhoea with bloating, abdominal cramps and flatus
Skin nodules
Disseminated fat necrosis – rare

INVESTIGATIONS

FBC
Normal

U + Es
Normal

LFTs
Raised if concurrent liver disease or cholestasis, but otherwise normal

Amylase ↑ or normal later in the disease. No prognostic value
Lipase may be ↑ or normal

72 h faecal fat collection >20 g/24 h (normal <7 g/24 h)

Pancreatic exocrine function tests
Lundh test – stimulation of pancreatic exocrine function by a test meal, followed by endoscopic sampling of pancreatic fluid for trypsin and amylase. These are low in chronic pancreatitis.
PABA test is now rarely used – patient given bentiromide after a peptide load, which is normally cleaved by pancreatic chymotrypsin to free PABA which is absorbed and excreted in the urine. PABA excretion is reduced in chronic pancreatitis, but this is dependent on other factors such as renal function.

Ultrasound
Abdominal ultrasound may show focal or diffuse enlargement, ductal irregularity and dilatation and pseudocysts (sensitivity 60–70%).
Endoscopic ultrasound is increasing in use. Can also perform fine needle aspiration by this method.
Magnetic resonance cholangiopancreatography (MRCP) is

non-invasive, but as yet lacks the sensitivity of ERCP.

DIAGNOSIS

Plain abdominal film may show pancreatic intraductal calcification in 30% (especially alcohol induced)
Abdominal CT has specificity of 90%
ERCP is useful to confirm the diagnosis.

DIFFERENTIAL DIAGNOSIS

Pancreatic malignancy is the major differential
Coeliac disease
Crohn's disease

Also consider:

Other malignancy
Other causes of malabsorption, e.g. bacterial overgrowth
Gallstones
Peptic ulcer disease
Irritable bowel syndrome
Endometriosis

COMPLICATIONS

Pancreatic pseudocyst formation. Cause of 5–10% of deaths with chronic pancreatitis due to complications of mechanical obstruction, erosion into blood vessels and infection. If small they require no treatment, but if larger may require percutaneous aspiration or surgery.

Abscess formation
Gastrointestinal bleeding

Mechanical obstruction to duodenum – pain after eating and early satiety.
   Mechanical obstruction to common bile duct – pain and jaundice with abnormal liver function tests.
   Pancreatic fistulae with ascites or a pleural effusion (these exudates have very high amylase levels).
   Splenic vein thrombosis with portal hypertension – may require splenectomy.
   Pseudo-aneurysm formation involving the splenic artery – treat with coil embolization if possible.

TREATMENT

Stop alcohol – improves prognosis, but may not affect pain
Pain control – beware problems of addiction to opiates
Intravenous vitamin supplementation
Oral pancreatic enzyme supplements – this often improves pain by diminishing the stimulation of cholecystokinin
Diet, oral hypoglycaemics and insulin may be required in the treatment of diabetes
Coeliac plexus nerve block may be considered, but side effects include postural hypotension, diarrhoea and paraparesis
Surgery is controversial. It has been used for pancreatic resection, and ductal drainage procedures. Surgery may also be indicated for drainage of larger pancreatic pseudocysts

Endoscopic treatments include sphincterotomy, pancreatic duct stent placement, stone extraction and pseudocyst drainage.

QUESTION SPOTTING

Grey case
More suited for this style of question. The question is unlikely to include all three of alcohol abuse, abdominal pain and raised amylase. A question with abdominal pain, weight loss and nausea/vomiting is likely to raise the suspicion of abdominal malignancy, but chronic pancreatitis should also be considered. Plain abdominal radiographs are easy to do and if they show pancreatic calcification the diagnosis is made. Abdominal CT will show this calcification and should pick up pancreatic or other abdominal malignancy.

Data interpretation
Interpretation of 3 day faecal fat excretion or pancreatic function test may suggest the diagnosis of chronic pancreatitis. Faecal fat levels tend to be much higher than for malabsorption syndromes such as coeliac disease.

RENAL DISEASE

4

HAEMOLYTIC URAEMIC SYNDROME AND THROMBOTIC THROMBOCYTOPENIC PURPURA

A syndrome comprising microangiopathic haemolysis, renal failure, thrombocytopenia, thought to be due to endothelial cell dysfunction. A variety of insults may trigger the syndrome.

With diarrhoeal prodrome
E. coli 0157, *Shigella*, *Yersinia* spp. (all produce Shiga toxin)

Without diarrhoeal prodrome
Viral or pneumococcal URTI
HIV
Idiopathic; may be familial
Pregnancy/postpartum
Malignant hypertension
Renal transplant
Other glomerulonephritis
SLE
Scleroderma
Drugs, including OCP, cyclosporin, mitomycin C, 5-fluorouracil, ticlopidine

NB. TTP follows a relapsing course in 10% of cases

SYMPTOMS

Bloody diarrhoea one week prior to onset
Tiredness, SOB (due to anaemia)
Nausea, vomiting, itching (due to uraemia)
Occasionally macroscopic haematuria

Neurological deficits
Are uncommon in HUS, but are common in TTP and include:

Seizures
Psychosis
Focal deficits; may be transient or permanent
Hallucinations

SIGNS

Pale (anaemia)
If onset is insidious, may see raised BP, hypertensive retinopathy
Asterixis (uraemia)
Fever
Purpuric rash

INVESTIGATIONS

FBC
Hb ↓
WCC ↑
Platelets ↓

U + Es
Na may be ↓ in ARF
K usually ↑
Urea and creatinine ↑

LFTs
Bilirubin ↑
Albumin ↓

Haptoglobins ↓ or absent
Reticulocytes ↑
Coombs' test negative
Urate ↑
LDH ↑
INR and APTT normal
Fibrin degradation products usually ↑
Blood film shows schistocytes and spherocytes

CT of the brain may show areas of infarction, or less commonly haemorrhage, in TTP

DIAGNOSIS

Renal biopsy shows thrombosis and necrosis of intrarenal vessels. This finding, together with renal failure and a microangiopathic haemolytic anaemia, thrombocytopenia plus normal coagulation, is strongly suggestive of HUS.

Gum biopsy or rectal biopsy may show microthrombi within the capillary bed in TTP.

DIFFERENTIAL DIAGNOSIS

Vasculitis
Malignant hypertension
Carcinomatosis
Septicaemia with DIC (clotting is abnormal)
Ischaemic colitis or ulcerative colitis
Haemorrhagic fevers, including Dengue
Malaria
Snake bite
SBE especially on prosthetic valves
HELLP syndrome (pregnancy) and pre-eclampsia

Evans syndrome (ITP + autoimmune haemolytic anaemia)
AV malformations

COMPLICATIONS

Bowel perforation/infarction may occur
GI bleeding
Pancreatitis
Acute coronary ischaemia
Myocarditis occurs rarely

TREATMENT

HUS

Supportive treatment includes correcting hypovolaemia, hyperkalaemia and anaemia. Dialysis is often necessary.

Steroids are widely used but have not been proven to affect outcome.

Plasma exchange is also used, but its efficacy is unclear at present.

Likewise, the benefit of using heparin or prostacyclins is also unproven.

TTP

Plasma exchange against FFP is the treatment of choice; this has been shown to reduce mortality. Some patients appear to improve on steroids; use of steroids may reduce the chance of relapse. Platelet transfusion is contraindicated as it can worsen the disease.

PROGNOSIS

Highly variable for HUS. Children tend to recover renal function more often than adults, and those with acute forms and/or diarrhoeal prodromes also seem to recover renal function more often than patients with a more insidious onset of disease.

Historical mortality for TTP is 90%. Treated mortality is around 10%.

QUESTION SPOTTING

Grey case

A 'classic' presentation involves a diarrhoeal prodrome, followed by:

Renal failure
Microangiopathic haemolytic anaemia
Thrombocytopenia
Normal clotting

In such a case, the major differential diagnosis is TTP which more commonly has neurological manifestations, and less commonly produces renal failure. The diseases are thought to be two ends of a spectrum of microthrombotic disease however.

HUS may occur without an obvious prodrome, and may have an insidious onset.

Data interpretation

Unlikely to appear in this section.

RENAL TRANSPLANT FAILURE

Renal transplants may fail for the same reasons as native kidneys, or for reasons specific to transplanted kidneys. Causes include

Pre-renal
Sepsis
Dehydration
Haemorrhage
Myocardial failure

Intrinsic renal failure
Arterial thrombosis
Venous thrombosis
Acute tubular necrosis
Infection
Rejection (hyperacute, acute or chronic)
Cyclosporin A toxicity
Relapse of original renal disease, especially focal segmental glomerulosclerosis, but also membranous, IgA, mesangiocapillary and anti-GBM disease
Renal artery stenosis
New glomerulonephritis, including CMV infection

Post-renal
Bladder outflow obstruction
Ureteric obstruction (e.g. from a lymphocoele, ureteric stenosis, clot in ureter)

CLINICAL FEATURES

Arterial thrombosis
Abrupt loss of graft function (anuria, biochemical derangement)
Often no other signs, but may be hypertensive if subtotal thrombosis
Occurs in first few days after transplant

Venous thrombosis
Occurs days to weeks after transplant
Loss of function (oliguria/anuria)
Painful, swollen graft
May have swollen ipsilateral leg
Graft occasionally ruptures, leading to haemorrhagic shock

Ureteric obstruction
Reduced graft function (oliguria/anuria)
Graft may slowly increase in size
Ipsilateral leg may swell (iliac vein compression)

Cyclosporin A toxicity
Reduced graft function
Improves when drug dose is reduced
Usually hypertensive (but this is often the case when cyclosporin A dose is in the therapeutic range)

Hyperacute rejection
Occurs within minutes of graft being perfused
Graft fails to work at all

Acute rejection
Most often occurs in first 3 to 6 months after transplant
Fever
Painful, swollen graft
Reduced function (oliguria/anuria)
Features may be less dramatic when taking cyclosporin

Chronic rejection
Usually asymptomatic; may present with symptoms of uraemia. There is usually no pain, swelling or fever

Infection
Painful, swollen graft
Fever, rigors
Dysuria and frequency
Reduced graft function

INVESTIGATIONS

FBC
Hb $\downarrow$ in chronic failure
WCC $\uparrow$ in sepsis, acute rejection. This response may be attenuated by azathioprine
Platelets usually normal

U + Es
Na may be $\downarrow$ in acute failure
K may be $\uparrow$

Urea and creatinine are $\uparrow$ in any form of transplant failure. It is important to know the baseline level however.

LFTs
Usually normal, but may be mildly $\uparrow$ (from azathioprine)
Calcium low or normal

ESR, CRP are raised in sepsis, acute rejection and recurrent vasculitis

Coagulation screen usually normal

PO_4 raised in transplant failure, especially if chronic

Urinalysis

Blood and protein in arterial or venous thrombosis, infection, acute rejection or some forms of vasculitis.

Protein only in chronic rejection or some forms of recurrent renal disease. Mild proteinuria also occurs in cyclosporin A toxicity.

Early acute rejection may show decreased urinary Na, increased urinary creatinine, proteinuria and so-called 'activated cells' in the urine sediment.

DIAGNOSIS

Renal U/S with doppler flow; this will diagnose obstruction to urine outflow, arterial and venous thrombosis and lymphocoele.

MSU for infection.

Cyclosporin A levels for potential toxicity.

Renal biopsy; can show acute or chronic rejection, or recurrent glomerulonephritis/other renal disease. Acute rejection produces interstitial oedema, with a lymphocytic infiltrate and evidence of vascular injury.

DIFFERENTIAL DIAGNOSIS

For a slow rise in urea or creatinine
Recurrence of original renal disease
Cyclosporin A toxicity
Chronic rejection
Also consider other nephrotoxic drugs, e.g. antibiotics, diuretics, ACE inhibitors

Fever, pain, swelling and rising creatinine
Acute rejection
Sepsis including UTI
Pre-renal causes
Venous thrombosis

TREATMENT

Acute rejection: antithymocyte immunoglobulin plus high dose methylprednisolone
Pre-renal failure; ensure good fluid loading and treat the cause
Recurrence of original renal disease: may need increased immunosuppression
Cyclosporin A toxicity: reduce dose
UTI: treat with antibiotics
Chronic rejection: No useful therapy at present

QUESTION SPOTTING

Grey case
You will usually be told that a transplant is present; if not, the iliac fossa mass is the clue.

Transplant failure is evidenced by a rising creatinine, which may be accompanied by oliguria or anuria.

Remember that transplant failure may not be due to rejection.

Remember that other opportunistic infections affect immunosuppressed transplant patients (e.g. TB, PCP, candida, CMV).

Data interpretation
Less likely to crop up in this section.

AMYLOIDOSIS

Deposition of fibrillar amyloid protein in target organs, which can include almost any organ in the body. Several types of amyloid are recognized, including AL (derived from Ig light chains), AA (derived from amyloid protein A, an acute phase reactant), and ATTR, derived from a mutant transthyretin protein.

CAUSES OF AMYLOIDOSIS

AL
Myeloma
Waldenström's macroglobulinemia
Non-Hodgkin's lymphoma
Other monoclonal gammopathies

AA
Any longstanding infection or inflammation, including:

Tuberculosis
Bronchiectasis
Osteomyelitis
Infected ulcers or burns
Whipple's disease
Leprosy

Rheumatoid arthritis
Behçet's disease
Adult Still's disease
Ankylosing spondylitis
Reiter's disease
Crohn's disease (rare in UC)
Familial Mediterranean fever
Renal cell carcinoma
Hodgkin's disease
Renal dialysis

CLINICAL FEATURES (AL amyloid)

Skin
Purpura, easy bruising. Amyloid plaques

Cardiac
Restrictive cardiomyopathy – tiredness, SOB, nausea. Right-sided signs more prominent
Conduction problems/heart block

Renal
Nephrotic syndrome, chronic renal failure: oedema, pruritus, anaemia.

Usually normotensive
Kidneys enlarged and may be palpable

Hepatic/GI
Hepatomegaly
Diarrhoea, constipation, early satiety, dysphagia
Malabsorption

Lung
Usually asymptomatic, but lung function changes seen.

Neurological
Sensory neuropathy: distal > proximal. Motor neuropathy is rare, as is CNS involvement.

Prominent autonomic features, especially postural hypotension.

Other
Hyposplenism in 24%. Splenomegaly in 5%
Lymphadenopathy is usually absent
Macroglossia (20%)
Nail dystrophy
Shoulder pad sign, polyarthropathy
Hypothyroidism (20%). Hypoadrenalism

Differences for AA amyloid
Cardiac involvement is rare
No macroglossia
Splenomegaly is more common
Gut involvement is usually asymptomatic

Differences with ATTR amyloid
Neurological dysfunction common
No macroglossia
Renal disease is mild
Cardiomyopathy less prominent, but conduction system problems are common

INVESTIGATIONS

FBC
Hb ↓ in renal failure
WCC normal
Platelets normal

U + Es
Na ↓ in hypoadrenalism
Urea, creatinine ↑ (renal impairment)

LFTs
Bilirubin usually normal
ALT usually normal

ALP $\downarrow$
Albumin $\downarrow$

ESR, CRP reflect underlying disease
Clotting occasionally deranged (due to binding
of clotting factors to amyloid or severe liver
disease)
Immunoglobulins may show monoclonal band in
AL amyloid
TFTs may show low T_4, raised TSH (if thyroid
involved)
Blood film may show Howell-Jolly bodies
(hyposplenism)

Urine shows proteinuria. May show Bence-Jones
proteins (AL)

ECG: may show poor R wave progression,
conduction delays/block

Echo: may show diastolic ventricular impairment
(restrictive), bright echo pattern to
myocardium

PFTs show reduced Kco

Chest X-ray may show pleural effusions and
reticulo-nodular shadowing

DIAGNOSIS

Rectal, fat or target organ biopsy. All have
70–80% sensitivity. Amyloid stains red with
Congo Red, and shows apple-green birefringence
under polarized light.

Diagnosis of AL amyloid
Monoclonal Ig or Bence-Jones protein in 90%
Monoclonal plasma cells on bone marrow biopsy

Diagnosis of ATTR amyloid
Isoelectric focusing of plasma to identify mutant
transthyretin protein.

TREATMENT

Avoid calcium channel blockers and digoxin if
cardiac involvement (may worsen condition).
    Restrictive cardiomyopathy may require
warfarin.
    Colchicine is effective in FMF amyloid.
    Chemotherapy can prolong life in AL amyloid,
but is poorly tolerated if cardiac involvement is
present.
    Liver transplant is the treatment of choice for
ATTR amyloid.

PROGNOSIS

One to two years for AL amyloid. Median
survival 6 months if cardiac involvement
Up to 15 year survival from diagnosis in ATTR
amyloid
Prognosis is dependent on the underlying disease
in AA amyloid

QUESTION SPOTTING

Grey case
The combination of hepatomegaly with or
without splenomegaly plus renal impairment
is a strong pointer to amyloidosis. Mention
of a large tongue should also make one
consider the diagnosis as should autonomic
neuropathy.

Data interpretation
Proteinuria and renal impairment in a patient
with an underlying inflammatory disorder should
prompt consideration of amyloid.

RENAL CELL CARCINOMA

Renal cell adenocarcinoma (hypernephroma) is derived from proximal tubular epithelial cells. Bilateral tumours occur in 1%. 25% present with metastases, usually to bone, lung or liver.

SYMPTOMS

Haematuria (65%)
Loin pain (20–40%)
Weight loss
Anorexia
Fevers/sweats (20%)
Left-sided scrotal swelling

SIGNS

Fever
Mass in flank (6–50%)
Hypertension (12%)
Left-sided varicocele

INVESTIGATIONS

FBC
Hb ↑ in 4% (erythropoietin production). ↓ in 35% (reduced erythropoietin)
WCC usually normal
Platelets usually normal; ↑ in 11%

U + Es
Usually normal

LFTs
May be ↑ if liver metastases. ALP may be ↑ if bony metastases or if reactive hepatitis present. Bilirubin usually normal.

Calcium may be ↑
ESR often ↑ (40%)

Chest X-ray may show 'cannonball' metastases.
Urine often shows haematuria. Does not usually contain malignant cells.

DIAGNOSIS

U/S, IVU or CT abdomen; angiography may also help to delineate tumour.

DIFFERENTIAL DIAGNOSIS

Other causes of haematuria
Other causes of a PUO
Rarer mesenchymal renal tumours
Xanthogranulomatous pyelonephritis
Renal cysts

COMPLICATIONS

Amyloidosis (3–5%)
Reactive hepatitis (4%) with hepatomegaly

TREATMENT

Surgery for non-metastatic tumours. Removal of the primary tumour may sometimes lead to regression of metastases.
Chemotherapy is used experimentally; a few tumours also respond to medroxyprogesterone.
Radiotherapy can be used in a neoadjuvant setting or for palliative reasons.

PROGNOSIS

50% 10 year survival for tumours confined to one kidney
5% 10 year survival for metastatic disease

QUESTION SPOTTING

Grey case
May present as a non-specific illness involving weight loss, fever, raised ESR; there is usually another clue to the diagnosis, e.g. haematuria or raised Hb +/– raised calcium.
You are unlikely to be told about a mass in the flank!

Data interpretation
As above. The Hb and calcium levels are the clues, along with a raised ESR.

RENAL TUBULAR ACIDOSIS (RTA)

Failure of the kidney to create acid urine by either distal tubular failure to exchange Na^+ for H^+ leading to excess bicarbonate in the filtrate; or the proximal tubule failure to excrete hydrogen ions. An important cause of normal anion gap acidosis.

There are four types:

TYPE I – DISTAL RTA

Distal RTA is the most common type. The disease presents at any age.

Causes

Congenital
Autosomal dominant, recessive and sex-linked all documented

Acquired
Autoimmune ($\uparrow$ immunoglobulin), e.g. Sjögren's syndrome, chronic active hepatitis, cryoglobulinaemia.
Nephrocalcinosis, e.g. hyperparathyroidism, excess vitamin D, medullary sponge kidney.
Drugs, e.g. amphotericin, lithium, analgesics.
Renal disease, e.g. transplanted kidney, obstructive uropathy, chronic pyelonephritis, sickle cell disease.

Symptoms
Anorexia
Fatigue
Renal colic from stones
Polyuria and polydipsia
Bone pain and weakness (due to osteomalacia caused by calcium loss in the urine and calcium from bone buffering excess H^+)
Constipation
Recurrent urinary tract infections secondary to renal stones
Renal failure

Investigations

FBC
Normal

U + Es
Na normal
K $\downarrow$
Urea and creatinine normal

Cl $\uparrow$
pH $\downarrow$
HCO^{3-} < 21 mmol/L

Urinalysis
urinary pH never < 5.5
urine ammonia $\downarrow$
urine calcium $\uparrow$ and urine citrate $\downarrow$ which leads to the formation of renal stones in the presence of an alkaline urine

Treatment
Treatment of underlying condition if possible
Sodium bicarbonate supplements
Potassium supplements
Citrate supplements
Thiazide diuretics may reduce plasma volume and thus increase proximal bicarbonate reabsorption
Vitamin D if osteomalacia

TYPE II – PROXIMAL RTA

Causes

Congenital
Hereditary – autosomal dominant
Cystinosis
Wilson's disease
Galactosaemia
Von Gierke's disease
Lowe's syndrome
Hereditary fructose intolerance

Acquired
Autoimmune with $\uparrow$ immunoglobulins, e.g. Sjögren's syndrome
Drugs, e.g. acetazolamide, lead, tetracyclines
Dysproteinaemic states, e.g. myeloma
Others, e.g. hyperparathyroidism, amyloid, nephrotic syndrome

Type II RTA is less common than type I. It most commonly occurs as part of a generalized proximal tubular defect that results in glycosuria, aminoaciduria, phosphaturia and renal tubular acidosis – the Fanconi syndrome.

The defect is a failure to secrete H^+ from the proximal tubule. This means that too much bicarbonate is left in the filtrate for the distal tubule to reabsorb. As the plasma bicarbonate falls, so the filtered bicarbonate load falls until the distal tubule is able to reabsorb all the bicarbonate and homeostasis is restored (at a plasma bicarbonate level of approx. 12–15 mmol/L). Because of the failure of the Na^+/H^+ pump in the proximal tubule, there is Na^+ wasting, causing polyuria and hypotension. This stimulates aldosterone secretion and the resulting Na^+/K^+ exchange causes hypokalaemia.

Renal calculi are not a feature. Rickets/osteomalacia are seen, but only as a failure of vitamin D metabolism which is often part of the Fanconi syndrome and are not due to calcium buffering.

Symptoms
Polyuria and polydipsia
Muscle weakness – rare. Caused by
    hypokalaemic myopathy
Bone pain from osteomalacia – rare

Investigations

FBC
Normal

U + Es
Na normal
$K \downarrow$
Urea and creatinine normal
$Cl \uparrow$

pH normal or $\downarrow$
Bicarbonate $\downarrow$
Ca may be $\downarrow$

Urinalysis
Urinary calcium normal
Glucose +
Protein +
Aminoaciduria +
pH normal

Treatment
Treatment of underlying condition if possible.
    Sodium bicarbonate supplements – huge doses may be required to overcome the 'leak'.
    Potassium citrate as required.

TYPE III

A combination of type I and type II and incredibly rare, so will not be covered here.

TYPE IV – HYPO-RENINAEMIC HYPOALDOSTERONISM

Probably the commonest of the renal tubular acidoses. Patients are acidotic and have hyperkalaemia.

Causes
Chronic tubulo-interstitial disease, e.g. reflux
    nephropathy
Diabetes mellitus leading to a failure of renin
    production
Primary adrenal disease, e.g. Addison's disease
Hereditary inborn errors of steroid synthesis –
    rare

The defect is caused either by hypoaldosteronism, or renal resistance to the effects of aldosterone. This reduces the capacity of the distal nephron to secrete H^+. Hyperkalaemia is directly due to loss of aldosterone action. This causes suppression of renal production of NH_4^+ which exacerbates the acidosis. The condition is more commonly seen in patients on prostaglandin inhibitors such as NSAIDs as renin production is partly dependent on prostaglandin synthesis.

Symptoms
Polyuria and polydipsia
Loin pain if reflux nephropathy

Investigations

FBC
Normal

U + Es
Na normal ($\downarrow$ if Addison's)
$K \uparrow$
Urea and creatinine normal
$pH \downarrow$
Bicarb $\downarrow$
Ca normal

Treatment
If significant acidosis or hyperkalaemia, treat
    with fludrocortisone

QUESTION SPOTTING

Grey case
May present with non-specific symptoms of polyuria and polydipsia, along with renal stones

or osteomalacia. These features should alert you to the possibility of renal tubular acidosis.

Data interpretation

This disorder is ideal for data interpretation questions. If given enough information in the question, always work out the anion gap.

Anion gap = $(Na + K) - (Cl + HCO_3)$.

Normal range = 10–18 mmol/L

If the anion gap is high in the presence of an acidosis, this means that there is an increased amount of an unmeasured anion, such as lactic acid or exogenous acid.

If the anion gap is normal in the presence of an acidosis, this means that HCl is being retained or HCO_3 is being lost.

There are a number of causes for each type:

Normal anion gap acidosis

GI bicarbonate loss by ileostomy or by
    diarrhoea, e.g. cholera diarrhoea
Renal tubular acidosis types I, II, IV
Cystectomy with implantation of ureters

Acetazolamide therapy
Pancreatic loss of HCO_3 via a pancreatic fistula
Ammonium chloride ingestion
Increased catabolism of lysine or arginine

High anion gap acidosis

Ketoacidosis
Insulin deficiency
Excess alcohol ingestion
Starvation

Lactic acidosis
Type A – poor tissue perfusion often with hypoxia occurs in shock (septic, hypovolaemic or cardiogenic), post seizure, severe hypoxia, and carbon monoxide poisoning.

Type B – reduced hepatic metabolism of lactic acid that may occur in diabetic ketoacidosis, metformin excess, haematological malignancies, hepatic failure, and alcohol excess.

Exogenous acids
Salicylate overdose
Ethylene glycol or methanol ingestion

BARTTER'S SYNDROME AND RELATED DISORDERS

Bartter's syndrome is caused by a defect in one of three ion channels in the thick ascending loop of Henle, the Na/K/2Cl channel (site of action of loop diuretics) being the prototypical mutant site. A closely related disorder, Gitelman's syndrome, is caused by mutations in the thiazide sensitive Na/Cl transporter in the distal convoluted tubule. Both these conditions may be mimicked by diuretic abuse or by rare autoimmune disorders affecting the aforementioned transporters.

SYMPTOMS

Polyhydramnios in utero (Bartter's only)
Weakness
Muscle cramps
Polyuria

SIGNS

BP is usually normal with no postural drop

INVESTIGATIONS

FBC
Usually normal

U + Es
Na usually normal
K invariably $\downarrow$
Urea and creatinine usually normal

LFTs
Usually normal

ESR usually normal unless other autoimmune disorders.
Bicarbonate usually $\uparrow$ (metabolic alkalosis)
Plasma renin $\uparrow$
Plasma aldosterone $\uparrow$

Urine
Urinary Na $\uparrow$
Urinary K $\uparrow$
Urinary Cl $\uparrow$
Urinary protein < 300 mg/24 h
Urine microscopy normal

DIAGNOSIS

1) Exclude diuretic abuse by repeated urine sampling for diuretics.

2) Bartter's syndrome typically shows hypercalciuria plus raised urinary prostaglandins. It is usually evident at birth or in early childhood.
3) Gitelman's syndrome typically shows hypocalciuria, hypomagnesemia plus raised urinary prostaglandins. It may not present until adulthood.
4) Immune related K^+ losing interstitial nephritis; suspect if other autoimmune phenomena present and urinary prostaglandins normal

Renal biopsy
Hyperplasia of the juxtaglomerular apparatus (JGA) is evident with Bartter's and Gitelman's syndromes.

COMPLICATIONS

Nephrocalcinosis due to chronic hypercalciuria

TREATMENT

Bartter's and Gitelman's: NSAIDs, K^+ supplements.

QUESTION SPOTTING

Grey case
Unlikely to appear in this section

Data interpretation
Good data interpretation cases. For all the above diagnoses, the clue is a hypokalaemic alkalosis with a normal blood pressure. A normal blood pressure argues against Cushing's or Conn's, and there is usually no history of vomiting, diarrhoea, fistulae or other drug ingestion.

The urine values show Na and K wasting with normal creatinine, pointing to a renal tubular problem.

Bartter's: tend to be young (<10 years), with high urinary calcium.

Gitelman's: tend to be adults, with low urinary calcium.

Diuretic abuse: suspect if a member of nursing staff, or job is allied to medicine.

Autoimmune: suspect if other features of autoimmune disease.

GOODPASTURE'S SYNDROME

An autoimmune disease which is characterized by deposition of antibodies against the glomerular basement membrane (anti-GBM antibodies) in various tissues, typically the lungs and kidneys. Due to different specificities of these antibodies, the disease may present in a variety of ways, and may not always present with the most typical features of haemoptysis and glomerulonephritis.

The incidence is bimodal with peaks at 30 (more men) and 60 (more women). The disease more typically presents in spring and this may be related to associated infection. Inhalation of hydrocarbons is also thought to trigger the disease.

SYMPTOMS

Cough
Shortness of breath
Pulmonary haemorrhage – variable and more common in smokers
Haematuria

SIGNS

Rare
Hypertension is not usually a feature

Note that systemic features of fever, rash, myalgia, malaise, headaches, joint pains and weight loss are not common but may occur. Chest pain and pleurisy is rare, cf. pulmonary embolism.

INVESTIGATIONS

FBC
Hb ↓ (MCV ↓ with prolonged haemoptysis due to iron deficiency)
WCC normal or ↑
Platelets normal or ↑

U + Es
Na normal
K normal or ↑ (with renal failure)
Urea ↑ with renal impairment
Creatinine ↑ with renal impairment

LFTs
Albumin ↓

ANCA may be positive in 30%. Usually pANCA.
ANA negative

Urinalysis
Dysmorphic red cells with red cell casts very common
Proteinuria is also common though not usually in the nephrotic range

Chest X-ray
Patchy shadows of intra-alveolar blood typically spreading out from the hilum. May be single or multiple. Shadows resolve within 2 weeks if no further bleeding.

Lung function tests
Increased CO transfer typical of pulmonary haemorrhage
A restrictive defect may occur with progressive disease

DIAGNOSIS

Anti GBM antibodies positive (usually IgG but may be IgA or IgM). False negative rate of 5–10%.

Renal biopsy
Linear immunofluorescence with rapidly progressive glomerulonephritis (RPGN) or crescentic glomerulonephritis. Linear staining occurs in Goodpasture's, SLE and diabetes. Anti-GBM antibodies may be demonstrated bound to renal tissue even if absent from plasma.

DIFFERENTIAL DIAGNOSIS

Renal/pulmonary syndromes may be seen in
SLE
Wegener's granulomatosis
Systemic sclerosis
Rheumatoid arthritis
Other systemic vasculitis: PAN, Churg-Strauss, Behçet's, giant cell arteritis, cryoglobulinaemia
Infection: TB, *Legionella*

Others: TTP and HUS, malignancy with glomerulopathy.

TREATMENT

Plasma exchange
Pulsed methylprednisolone

These two therapies are the only truly effective therapies. Prednisolone is rarely effective in the acute phase but tends to be used in conjunction with cytotoxics such as cyclophosphamide or azathioprine to prevent rebound after the plasma exchange.

Transplantation is now increasingly used. Goodpasture's may recur in the transplanted kidney, but this is usually a milder form (possibly due to time delay from initial onset of disease, and due to the immunosuppressive regimen).

PROGNOSIS

Generally poor despite treatment if advanced renal disease. Although anti-GBM antibody titres show poor correlation with prognosis, patients with high ANCA but low anti-GBM titres tend to do well, but show relapses which do not tend to occur in ANCA negative patients.

QUESTION SPOTTING

Grey case

The typical patient is a young white male smoker who presents with haemoptysis. Anti-GBM antibodies with renal biopsy should be diagnostic but look to exclude other conditions seen in the differential like SLE.

Data interpretation

You may be asked to interpret a renal biopsy in the setting of a patient with rapidly progressive glomerulonephritis. This occurs in Goodpasture's, SLE, Wegener's, cryoglobulinaemia, Henoch-Schönlein purpura, PAN, as well as the typical post infections, and idiopathic types. Think of Goodpasture's if asked to interpret lung function tests with raised Kco.

RHEUMATOLOGICAL DISEASE

5

SYSTEMIC LUPUS ERYTHEMATOSUS

SLE is a multisystem autoimmune disorder of unknown aetiology, characterized by widespread derangement of humoral and cell mediated immunity. Vasculitis underlies many of the organ derangements. A minority of sufferers have mutations of complement components, especially C_1, C_2, C_4.

FEATURES (% = symptoms at onset of disease)

Joints
Arthralgia, arthritis (60%). Usually non-erosive, migratory. Effusions are uncommon. Jaccoud's arthropathy may develop.

Myalgia
Myositis (10%)

Skin (60%)
Raynaud's phenomenon (25%)
Livedo reticularis
Photosensitive rashes, e.g. butterfly rash
Urticaria
Purpura
Discoid lesions (may occur alone)
Alopecia

Renal (25%)
Glomerulonephritis
Vasculopathy with hypertension

Neurological (20%)
Psychosis
Fits
Headaches
Memory impairment
Cranial nerve palsies
Aseptic meningitis
Peripheral neuropathy

Cardiac
Endocarditis (Libman-Sacks)
Pericarditis
Myocarditis

Lung (5%)
Pleuritic pain; effusions are uncommon
Pneumonitis (acute or chronic)

GI (uncommon)
Pancreatitis
Peritonitis
Mesenteric vasculitis

Other
Hepatomegaly, splenomegaly
Lymphadenopathy (non-tender) (15%)
Arterial and venous thrombosis (due to antiphospholipid syndrome)
Weight loss

INVESTIGATIONS

FBC
Hb sometimes ↓ (haemolysis, chronic disease)
MCV normal (↑ in haemolysis)
WCC often ↓ (especially lymphocytes)
Platelets sometimes ↓
Reticulocytes ↑ in haemolysis

U + Es
Urea and creatinine ↑ in renal disease

LFTs
Bilirubin ↑ in haemolysis
ALT, ALP ↑ in active disease, especially after administration of salicylates

Haptoglobins absent in haemolysis
INR normal
APTT prolonged in antiphospholipid syndrome
ESR ↑
CRP usually normal; ↑ in serositis or concomitant disease, e.g. infection
CK ↑ in myositis
Igs ↑
Immune complexes ↑
C_3 ↓
C_4 ↓
Total complement activity ↓

Antibodies
ANA positive in 95%.
   dsDNA positive in 60%; high specificity for SLE.
   anti-Ro positive in 20–60%. Also positive in Sjögren's syndrome.
   anti-La positive in 15–40%. Also positive in Sjögren's syndrome.
   anti-Sm positive in 10–30%. High specificity for SLE.
   anti-RNP is a marker for mixed connective tissue disease.
   Rheumatoid factor positive in 25–50%.

VDRL often false positive (antiphospholipid syndrome).

Urine may show proteinuria, haematuria.

DIAGNOSIS

Four from the following must be present:

Malar (butterfly) rash
Discoid rash
Photosensitivity
Oral ulcers
Arthritis
Serositis (pleuritic, pericarditis)
Renal disease (>500 mg proteinuria/day, cellular casts)
Neurological disorder
Haematological disorder (low Hb, WCC or platelets)
Positive ANA
Immunological disorder (LE cells, anti-dsDNA, anti-Sm or false positive VDRL)

DIFFERENTIAL DIAGNOSIS

Autoimmune disease
Rheumatoid arthritis
Adult Still's disease
Mixed connective tissue disease
Systemic sclerosis
Polymyositis
Behçet's disease
Primary vasculitides
Primary antiphospholipid syndrome

Infections
Viral arthritis
Whipple's disease
SBE
Lyme disease
Syphilis
TB

Other
AIP
TTP/HUS
PNH
Drug reactions
Lymphoma
Sarcoidosis
Atrial myxoma

Inflammatory bowel disease
Familial Mediterranean fever

TREATMENT

Mild (skin and joints only)
Hydroxychloroquine
Topical steroids
Sun block

Moderate
Oral steroids
Azathioprine as a steroid sparing agent

Severe (progressive renal disease, neurological disease)
Cyclophosphamide, azathioprine
Steroids

COMPLICATIONS

Infections
End stage renal failure
Atherosclerosis
Pulmonary embolus
Osteonecrosis
Permanent neurological damage
Shrinking lung syndrome

PROGNOSIS

>90% 5 year survival
70% alive at 20 years

QUESTION SPOTTING

Grey case
SLE is the multisystem disorder par excellence. Clues to the diagnosis are:

Young female patient
Low WCC +/– low platelets
Renal disease
Rashes
High ESR with relatively normal CRP

Consider SLE whenever multiple organ systems are involved in a young woman and there is no immediately obvious cause or she has unexplained spontaneous abortions or neuropsychiatric illness.

Data interpretation
Less likely to crop up in this section.

RHEUMATOID ARTHRITIS

Unknown mechanism, but autoimmunity is the most likely. The trigger is thought to be T helper cell activation leading to production of pro-inflammatory mediators such as IL-1 and TNF-α. This in turn leads to persistent cellular activation, autoimmunity and inflammation. Tissue damage is caused by immune complex deposition and direct cell-mediated immunity. Inflammation of synovium causes thickening and effusions with joint and bone destruction.

1% of the population world-wide have rheumatoid arthritis. Male to female ratio 1 : 3. Peak incidence in 4th–5th decade, but can occur at any age. There is a family history in 5–10% patients.

Classical disease gives early morning stiffness and pain in a few peripheral joints initially, but disease can be highly variable.

Pattern of disease
Insidious (70%)
Acute (15%)
Systemic (10%)
Palindromic (5%)

CLINICAL FEATURES

Joints
Swelling
Pain
Stiffness (especially if joint inactive)
Reduced joint motion
Subluxation
Joint instability
Deformity
Contractures

Classical changes in the hands and feet include: ulnar deviation of fingers, swan neck deformities, Boutonnière deformity, Z deformity of thumbs, clawing of toes.

Tendonitis
Bursitis

Extra-articular

Systemic
Fever
Weight loss
Fatigue
Increased infection risk

Musculoskeletal
Muscle wasting

Haematological
Anaemia

Lymphatic
Splenomegaly
Lymphadenopathy (50%)

Skin
Nodules
Fistulae
Pyoderma gangrenosum
Ulcers

Neurological
Cervical cord compression secondary to
    atlanto-axial subluxation
Mononeuritis multiplex
Compression neuropathy esp. carpal tunnel
    syndrome
Peripheral neuropathy (sensorimotor)
Stroke

Ocular
Episcleritis
Scleritis
Scleromalacia
Keratoconjunctivitis sicca (10%)

Cardiovascular – rare except for pericarditis
Pericarditis causing effusions and sometimes
    pericardial constriction
Myocarditis
Endocarditis
Conduction abnormalities
Coronary vasculitis
Aortitis, arteritis

Pulmonary
Nodules – may cavitate
Effusions – v common: exudates with $\uparrow$ white
    cells, $\uparrow$ LDH, $\downarrow$ glucose, $\uparrow$ Rheumatoid
    factor, $\downarrow$ complement
Fibrosis – see Fig. 6
Bronchiolitis obliterans
Haemorrhage
Caplan's syndrome

Amyloid

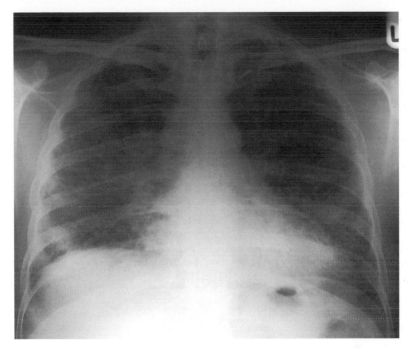

Fig. 6. Fibrosing alveolitis secondary to rheumatoid arthritis. This chest X-ray shows small lung volume for maximal inspiration. There is widespread reticular nodular shadowing in the mid and lower zones with a peripheral distribution. These appearances are typical for any fibrosing alveolitis, including cryptogenic, drug induced, and that secondary to connective tissue diseases.

INVESTIGATIONS

FBC

Hb ↓ (MCV normal, ↓ or ↑; sulphasalazine causes ↑ MCV)

WBC ↑ – if leucopenia and thrombocytopenia think of Felty's syndrome

Eosinophilia may occur

Platelets ↑

Hb may be ↓ due to:

1) Iron deficiency anaemia from NSAIDs
2) Folate deficiency (↑ cell turnover)
3) B12 deficiency due to pernicious anaemia
4) Chronic disease
5) Haemolytic anaemia
6) Aplastic anaemia secondary to drug therapy

U + Es

Na normal

K normal

Urea and creatinine ↑ if renal involvement or drug toxicity (NSAIDs, penicillamine, gold, cyclosporin A)

LFTs

May be raised with sulphasalazine or methotrexate

ESR ↑ may stay high even when disease not active

CRP ↑

Complement C_3 and C_4 ↓

Rheumatoid factor often positive (75%)

ANA may be positive (30%)

Cryoglobulins may be present

X-rays

Periarticular osteoporosis

Loss of joint space

Erosions

Subluxation and ankylosis

Joint aspiration

Yellow, cloudy, 2000–10000 cells/mm^3; predominantly neutrophils

DIFFERENTIAL DIAGNOSIS

Infective arthritis
Rheumatic fever
SLE
Adult Still's disease
Sero-negative arthritis such as psoriatic arthritis, ankylosing spondylitis, etc.

COMPLICATIONS

Amyloid
Lymphoma
Other malignancy

TREATMENT

Symptom relief
Suppression of disease process
Bed rest and physiotherapy
Rest splints
Simple analgesics, e.g. paracetamol, codeine, tramadol
Non steroidal anti-inflammatory drugs (NSAIDs)

Disease modifying drugs

Hydroxychloroquine
Sulphasalazine
Methotrexate
Penicillamine

Gold
Dapsone (Note: slow acetylators prone to haemolytic anaemia)

Systemic steroids – in severe exacerbation or severe extra-articular manifestations, e.g. scleritis.

Intra-articular steroids

Immunomodulation with azathioprine, cyclophosphamide, cyclosporin A, but only in severe disease where other therapies failed. Surgery for tendon repairs, synovectomy, soft tissue decompression, arthroplasty, joint replacement, arthrodesis.

PROGNOSIS

Variable. Worse if: high RF titre, insidious onset, continuous active disease without remission, nodules, erosions, extra-articular disease.

QUESTION SPOTTING

Grey case

Ideal for these questions. Multiple extra-articular manifestations make it easy to confuse with SLE, rheumatic fever.

Data interpretation

Less suited for this type of question, but you might be asked to interpret some lung function tests.

SYSTEMIC SCLEROSIS

An autoimmune disease of unknown aetiology which results in vascular damage and fibrosis in a number of organ systems. Various forms are recognized, including CREST syndrome, systemic sclerosis and morphoea. All forms are more common in women (3 : 1). CREST (limited disease) consists of:

Calcinosis
Raynaud's phenomenon
Oesophageal dysmotility
Sclerodactyly (usually limited to distal limbs)
Telangiectasia

CLINICAL FEATURES

Skin
Raynaud's phenomenon
Nailfold capillary abnormalities
Itching and oedema of skin
Thickened, waxy skin
Hyperpigmented or hypopigmented areas
Telangiectasia
Calcium deposits in skin

GI tract
Dysphagia
Dry mouth (sicca syndrome)
Restricted mouth opening
Nausea, anorexia (gastric paresis)
Malabsorption
Constipation +/– diarrhoea (hypomotility)
Pseudo-obstruction

Musculoskeletal
Arthritis
Tendonitis
Myositis

Renal
Hypertensive renal crisis with renal failure

Lung
Fibrosing alveolitis
Pulmonary vessel disease, leading to pulmonary hypertension

Cardiac
Cor pulmonale
Myocardial fibrosis: arrhythmias, heart block

Other
Impotence
Trigeminal neuralgia
Carpal tunnel syndrome
Sensorimotor neuropathy
Autonomic neuropathy
Dry eyes

Gut and pulmonary involvement may progress over a period of years

INVESTIGATIONS

FBC
Hb may be $\downarrow$
MCV normal
WCC usually normal
Platelets usually normal

U + Es
Urea and creatinine $\uparrow$ in renal disease
Calcium normal

LFTs
Abnormal in PBC
Bilirubin $\uparrow$ in haemolysis

TFTs may show hypothyroidism
CK $\uparrow$ in myositis
ESR often $\uparrow$
Cold agglutinins may be present
Blood film may show fragmented RBCs in hypertensive renal crises

Antibodies
ANA positive in 80–90%
Rheumatoid factor positive in 30–40%
Anticentromere is specific for CREST; 60% sensitivity
Scl-70 is specific for diffuse systemic sclerosis; 40% sensitivity
Antimitochondrial positive in 10–15%; increased chance of developing PBC

Hand X-rays show resorption of phalangeal tufts, calcinosis (see Fig. 7)
Chest X-ray may show basal fibrosis

PFTs
Reduced FVC
Restrictive pattern
Low Kco

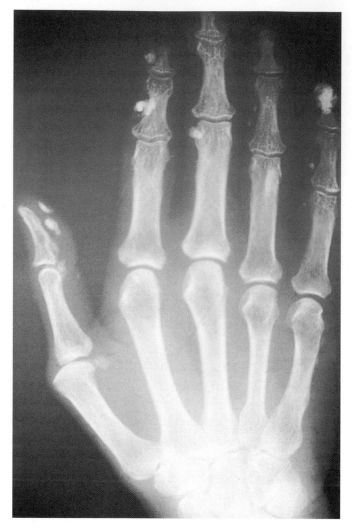

Fig. 7.   Scleroderma. This hand X-ray shows finger pulp calcinosis which is almost exclusive to scleroderma. There is also some evidence of tuft erosion to the terminal phalanx.

ECG may show evidence of heart block or conduction delay. LVH if hypertensive renal disease has been present for some time.

DIAGNOSIS

Is on clinical grounds; presence of Scl-70 or anti-centromere antibody is useful confirmation.

ASSOCIATIONS

Primary biliary cirrhosis in 3% of patients with CREST
Thyroid disease (especially hypothyroidism) in 20–40%

DIFFERENTIAL DIAGNOSIS

Sarcoidosis

Myxoedema
Chronic graft versus host disease
Overlap connective tissue disease
Porphyrias
Acromegaly

Also consider other causes of microangiopathy and other causes of pulmonary/renal syndromes (e.g. Wegener's, Goodpasture's, SLE).

TREATMENT

Hand care, hand warmers and calcium channel blockers for Raynaud's
Prostacyclin infusion for severe Raynaud's, renal disease and pulmonary hypertension
Prokinetic agents for dysmotility
Proton pump inhibitors for gastro-oesophageal reflux
ACE inhibitors for renal disease including hypertensive crises
Steroids, cyclophosphamide or azathioprine for pulmonary fibrosis

Surgery may help calcium deposits, and digital sympathectomy may aid pregangrenous digits

PROGNOSIS

5 year survival for diffuse disease is 40–75%

QUESTION SPOTTING

Grey case
Perhaps more likely to present as a complication in a patient known to have systemic sclerosis, e.g.
Renal hypertensive crisis
Lung fibrosis
PBC
Malabsorption

Data interpretation
As above.

WEGENER'S GRANULOMATOSIS

Vasculitis affecting small arteries in which granulomas are a feature, cf. polyarteritis nodosa.

The classical triad is:

upper respiratory tract granulomas
lower respiratory tract granulomas
necrotizing focal glomerulonephritis

Peak incidence in the 5th decade and more common in men. There is also a limited form with pure pulmonary disease and no damaging renal vasculitis.

CLINICAL FEATURES

General
Malaise
Arthralgia
Fever

Upper respiratory
Rhinitis
Epistaxis
Sinusitis
Serous otitis media
Nasal destruction leading to collapsed nasal
    bridge
Ulcers in palate, pharynx and sinuses

Lower respiratory
Note that there is often paucity of clinical signs
    despite florid radiographical changes
Cough
Haemoptysis
Chest pain
Dyspnoea
Bronchial obstruction causing atelectasis
Pleural involvement causing pleural effusions
    and pneumothorax

Renal
Glomerulonephritis – ranges from insidious to
    fulminant

Skin
Vasculitic rash – maculopapular or bullous. May
become necrotic.
    Nail fold infarcts.

Nervous system
Peripheral neuropathy including mononeuritis
    multiplex

Intracerebral granulomas

Eyes
Episcleritis
Scleritis
Uveitis
Retinal vasculitis
Optic neuritis
Optic pseudotumour causing proptosis

Cardiovascular
Pericarditis
Coronary arteritis

INVESTIGATIONS

FBC
Hb ↓ (MCV normal)
WCC ↑ (neutrophilia)
Platelets ↑

U + Es
Na normal
K normal (unless acute renal failure)
Urea and creatinine ↑

LFTs
Albumin ↓
Otherwise normal

CRP ↑
ESR ↑
cANCA positive (70–90%) (cytoplasmic ANCA
    against proteinase-3)
pANCA positive (5–10%) (perinuclear ANCA
    against myeloperoxidase)
Rheumatoid factor occasionally positive
ANA occasionally positive
Anti-GBM antibodies negative
Anti-smooth muscle antibodies occasionally
    positive
IgA ↑ or normal
IgG and IgM normal

Urinalysis
Blood + and red cell casts
Protein +

Chest X-ray
Typically multiple nodules (which may cavitate)
throughout both lung fields (see lung cancer for
differential). Nodules may reach several
centimetres in size, but rapidly resolve or evolve.

Evidence of pleural involvement with pleural effusions or rarely pneumothorax.

Bronchial obstruction may be seen as localised atelectasis.

DIAGNOSIS

Lung biopsy
Typical features include giant cells at the centre of a necrotic nodule with generalized arterial and venous inflammation. Upper airway histology is less specific.

Renal biopsy
Focal necrotizing glomerulonephritis with frequent crescent formation which is indistinguishable from Goodpasture's syndrome and Henoch-Schönlein syndrome.

DIFFERENTIAL DIAGNOSIS

See polyarteritis nodosa

Pulmonary-renal syndromes
Goodpasture's disease
Henoch-Schönlein syndrome
Churg-Strauss
Rheumatoid arthritis
SLE
Microscopic polyarteritis

TREATMENT

High dose steroids.
    Cyclophosphamide with MESNA.

Possible to switch to low dose azathioprine with low dose prednisolone for maintenance treatment.

Plasma exchange can help in severe or resistant disease. Likewise intravenous gamma globulin is also of use in difficult cases.

The limited form may sometimes be controlled by co-trimoxazole.

PROGNOSIS

80% 5 year survival

QUESTION SPOTTING

Grey case
An atypical history may be misleading and Wegener's may be difficult to distinguish from other forms of vasculitis. A raised WBC and platelets argues against SLE, and a positive cANCA (if given) will help the diagnosis. Churg-Strauss syndrome and microscopic polyarteritis may be positive for either pANCA or cANCA, but Churg-Strauss patients will be atopic, and microscopic polyarteritis does not involve the upper airway and the lung lesions do not cavitate.

The typical triad of upper and lower respiratory involvement and renal involvement should point to the diagnosis.

Data Interpretation
Less likely, but renal failure with markers of inflammation, together with a chest X-ray with (cavitating) nodules or a histology report may suggest Wegener's as a diagnosis.

POLYARTERITIS NODOSA

A necrotizing vasculitis of unknown aetiology, affecting medium to small sized arteries and leading to occlusion and aneurysm formation. It is associated with a number of other diseases, including hepatitis B and HIV infection. Granuloma formation is not a feature of the disease.

The disease typically affects middle aged/elderly men.

CLINICAL FEATURES

General
Fever
Tachycardia
Weight loss

Skin (50%)
Digital gangrene
Purpura
Livedo reticularis

Musculoskeletal
Myalgia (50%)
Arthralgia (50%)
Arthritis (20%)

Gastrointestinal (30%)
GI bleeding
Acute abdomen, e.g. RIF or RUQ pain
Mesenteric infarction

Cardiac
Hypertension (25%)
Pericarditis
MI (uncommon)

Renal
Chronic or acute renal failure
Glomerulonephritis (uncommon)

Hepatic
Hepatitis (uncommon)
Hepatic necrosis (uncommon)

Neurological
Mononeuritis multiplex (50–70%)
Stroke (uncommon)

Other
Pneumonitis (uncommon)
Retinal haemorrhage (uncommon)

INVESTIGATIONS

FBC
Hb ↓
MCV normal
WCC ↑
Platelets sometimes ↑

U + Es
Urea and creatinine often ↑

LFTs
ALP may be ↑ in liver involvement
Albumin ↓

Clotting usually normal
ESR ↑
CRP ↑
C_3, C_4 may be ↓
Total complement activity is ↓
Immune complexes often present
Rheumatoid factor occasionally positive
ANA negative
pANCA usually negative (see below)

Urine shows proteinuria and haematuria

DIAGNOSIS

The definition of polyarteritis nodosa changes every few years, particularly with respect to the dividing line between PAN and microscopic polyarteritis. Diagnosis is usually on clinical history, plus demonstration of
a) Aneurysms in medium sized vessels at angiography and/or
b) Necrotizing vasculitis in medium sized arteries on biopsy of an affected organ

In most cases of 'classical' PAN, pANCA is negative; however, it may be positive (10%) if small vessels are also involved.

DIFFERENTIAL DIAGNOSIS

Other primary vasculitides, e.g.
Wegener's granulomatosis
Microscopic polyarteritis

SLE
Rheumatoid arthritis
Buerger's disease
Ergotism
SBE

Atrial myxoma
Cryoglobulinaemia
TTP
Malignancy

TREATMENT

High dose corticosteroids, with additional cyclophosphamide especially if any evidence of small vessel involvement.

PROGNOSIS

60% 5 year survival with treatment

QUESTION SPOTTING

Grey case

Any organ dysfunction plus hypertension may be due to PAN, especially if there is evidence of glomerulonephritis or recurrent GI symptoms.

PAN is typically ANA and ANCA negative; these are the clues to differentiate it from other vasculitides.

Data interpretation

Less likely to crop up in this section.

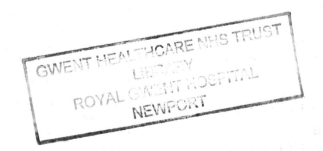

ADULT ONSET STILL'S DISEASE

A multisystem autoimmune disease of unknown aetiology. Onset is usually between ages 16 and 35. Females are affected nearly twice as often as males.

SYMPTOMS

Swinging pyrexia, often up to 40°C
Sore throat
Arthritis
Myalgia
Chest pain from pericarditis or pleurisy
Abdominal pain from peritoneal inflammation
Rash, usually maculopapular

SIGNS

Fever
Lymphadenopathy
Splenomegaly
Hepatomegaly
Abdominal tenderness

INVESTIGATIONS

FBC
Hb often ↓
WCC ↑, with neutrophilia
Platelets often ↑

U + Es
Usually normal

LFTs
Often raised; mild derangement
Albumin may be ↓

ESR invariably ↑
CRP ↑
Rheumatoid factor negative
Antinuclear antibody negative

X-rays show cartilage loss and joint erosions, most commonly in wrist and feet, but also in spine, shoulders, all finger joints.

Joint fluid shows neutrophil leucocytosis

DIAGNOSIS

All of the following must be present:
Arthritis for >6 weeks

$T > 39.5°C$
Negative rheumatoid factor
Negative ANA

Plus 2 of:
$WCC > 15 \times 10^9/L$
Macular/papular rash
Serositis
Hepatomegaly
Splenomegaly
Lymphadenopathy

DIFFERENTIAL DIAGNOSIS

Other causes of a PUO, especially:
Infections
Leukaemia
Lymphoma
Sarcoidosis
Endocarditis
Rheumatic fever
SLE (a few cases are ANA negative)

COMPLICATIONS

Rarely
Hepatic failure
Renal failure
Disseminated intravascular coagulation (DIC)
Myocarditis
Endocarditis
Amyloidosis

Extensive polyarticular destructive arthropathy may occur over time.

TREATMENT

High dose NSAIDs
Steroids for severe systemic disease

Disease modifying drugs (e.g. gold, cyclosporin) have been tried long term with some success.

PROGNOSIS

Occasional life threatening complications. Significant progressive, destructive polyarthritis in approximately 50%.

QUESTION SPOTTING

Grey case

Presents as:

Arthritis and pyrexia with negative ANA, ASOT
   and rheumatoid factor
An SLE like picture with negative ANA

Data interpretation

Less likely, but again, an arthritis with negative
autoimmune markers is the hallmark of adult
Still's disease.

PAGET'S DISEASE OF BONE

An increase in bone osteoclast activity, which leads to increased osteoblast activity. Bone turnover is thus increased, with areas of bone thickening and resorption. This weakens the bone, leading to fractures. The aetiology is unclear, but viral inclusion bodies have been found in osteoclasts. Prevalence in the UK is 3–9%, rising with age.

SYMPTOMS

Deafness
Bone pain
Bone deformity
Joint pain
Numbness/paraesthesia

SIGNS

Bony deformity
Warm bones
Reduced hearing acuity

Reduced sensation
Dermatomal from nerve root entrapment
Cord compression (rare)

Signs of cardiac failure (rare)

INVESTIGATIONS

FBC
Normal

U + Es
Normal

LFTs
ALP ↑ (bone isoenzyme)
GGT normal
Calcium normal unless immobile

ESR normal
Acid phosphatase may be ↑
PSA normal
PO_4 normal
PTH normal
Vitamin D normal

Urinary hydroxyproline ↑

X-rays
Expanded bone, coarse trabeculae
Areas of sclerosis and porosis
Axial skeleton most often affected
Periarticular calcification
Microfractures on convex surface of deformed bone

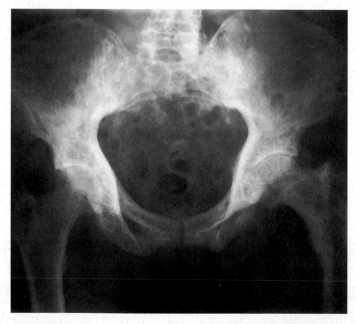

Fig. 8.   Paget's disease of bone. This pelvic X-ray shows very typical features of Paget's disease of bone. There is diffuse and severe sclerosis with coarse trabeculation and bony expansion. The disease is also apparent in the proximal femurs.

See skull and hip X-rays for typical examples
(Figs 8 and 9)
Bone scan shows greatly increased uptake in
affected areas

DIAGNOSIS

A typical X-ray appearance, especially in the
context of warm, deformed bones. Raised bony
ALP with normal calcium, PO_4 and vitamin D is
likely to be due to Paget's.

DIFFERENTIAL DIAGNOSIS

Metastatic malignancy (especially prostate)
Osteomalacia
Differential diagnosis of isolated raised ALP
Paget's disease of bone
Primary biliary cirrhosis
Hepatic metastatic malignancy

COMPLICATIONS

Increased risk of fracture
Osteoarthritis (especially of knee)
Osteogenic sarcoma (<1%)
High output cardiac failure in very extensive
disease
Cord compression
Nerve root entrapment
Cranial nerve palsies

TREATMENT

Bisphosphonates are the treatment of choice; IV
pamidronate is used if pressure symptoms are
present, otherwise oral bisphosphonates can be
used. Calcium and vitamin D may be needed to
prevent secondary hyperparathyroidism.
Calcitonin may be used as an adjunct to control
pain in the short term.

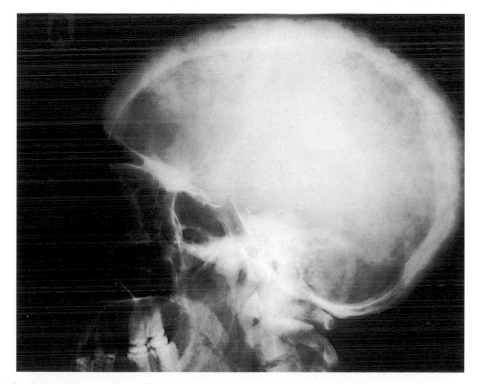

Fig. 9. Paget's disease of bone. The skull X-ray also shows typical features of Paget's disease of bone.

QUESTION SPOTTING

Grey case

Unlikely to occur, but just possible as part of a cord compression scenario. Look out for deafness plus non-specific aches and pains.

Data interpretation

A raised ALP with other bone markers normal and a normal GGT. Beware a slightly raised calcium may occur if the patient has been immobile due to their disease.

BEHÇET'S DISEASE

Behçet's disease is a multisystem vasculitic disease of unknown aetiology. It is thought to have an autoimmune basis, but infective triggers may also play a role. It is most common in peoples living along the Old Silk route, and is also common in the Japanese population.

CLINICAL FEATURES

Mouth ulcers
Dysuria
Dyspareunia (from genital ulcers)
Epididymitis

Skin lesions (75%)
Erythema nodosum
Acne
Papulopustular lesions

Eye lesions (50%)
Anterior uveitis (bilateral in 90%)
Choroidoretinitis
Keratitis
Conjunctivitis

Neurological (5–20%)
TIAs
Myelitis
Meningoencephalitis
Seizures
Psychosis
Sudden deafness
Pseudobulbar palsy

Arthritis (50%)
May follow any pattern, including sacroiliitis.
Usually non-erosive.

GI tract
Diarrhoea.
Rectal, intestinal and stomach ulcers

Cardiac (5–10%)
MI, myocardial ischaemia
Granulomatous endocarditis
Arrhythmias
Pericarditis

Rarer associations
Myositis
DVT, IVC/SVC thrombosis
Budd-Chiari syndrome
Arterial occlusion and aneurysms

Renal vein thrombosis
Pulmonary vasculitis
Amyloidosis (2%)
Lymphadenopathy

INVESTIGATIONS

FBC
Hb may be ↓
WCC mildly ↑ or normal
Platelets usually normal

U + Es
Usually normal

LFTs
Usually normal

ESR ↑
CRP ↑
C_3/C_4 normal or ↑
Immune complexes show modest ↑ in 50%
Rheumatoid factor negative
ANA negative
IgA often ↑
IgM, IgG levels are variable

DIAGNOSIS

Diagnostic criteria
Oral ulceration three times in 1 year plus two of:

Recurrent genital ulceration
Uveitis or retinal vasculitis
Skin lesions as described above
Positive pathergy test

Pathergy test: A sterile needle is used to produce a subcutaneous lesion, and the result read after 48 h. Presence of an erythematous papule >2 mm in diameter is considered a positive test.

The test is not specific; positive results are also seen in CML and spondyloarthropathies. The test is more likely to be positive in active disease and in certain populations.

DIFFERENTIAL DIAGNOSIS

Rheumatoid arthritis
Reiter's syndrome
Stevens-Johnson syndrome
Crohn's disease

Ulcerative colitis
Neurological lesions may mimic MS

TREATMENT

Eyes, skin: topical steroids
   Systemic steroids may be needed for internal disease; azathioprine or colchicine are also effective.
Thalidomide is useful for difficult to treat ulcers, and cyclosporin can be used for resistant uveitis.

PROGNOSIS

Disease runs a relapsing/remitting course. Prognosis is good unless neurological, pulmonary or vascular problems supervene.

QUESTION SPOTTING

Grey case

A clue to the diagnosis is often Turkish or Japanese origin of the patient. A combination of oral ulcers, genital ulcers and iritis suggests the diagnosis; if neurological symptoms are also present, the diagnosis becomes very likely (neurological symptoms should not occur in Crohn's or Reiter's).

Data interpretation

Unlikely to crop up in this section.

RELAPSING POLYCHONDRITIS

Relapsing polychondritis is a rare disease of uncertain aetiology, but probably an autoimmune reaction to collagen. Causes inflammation of tissues with high glycosaminoglycan content. This is mostly cartilage, but the disease can also affect the aortic valve, sclera, cornea and inner ear. The disease has a variable course, and is often episodic.

CLINICAL FEATURES

Ears
Bilateral auricular chondritis
Cochlear and vestibular damage leading to
  conduction deafness

Eyes
Ocular inflammation leading to uveitis, scleritis
  and episcleritis

Nose
Nasal chondritis causing a 'saddle nose'
  appearance

Joints
Non-erosive seronegative polyarthritis in up to
  60%

Respiratory
Laryngeal and tracheal cartilage collapse,
  leading to respiratory obstruction
Hoarse voice
Throat pain

Cardiac
Aortic root dilatation
Aortic regurgitation
Conduction defects
Aneurysms
Systemic vasculitis

Skin
Erythema nodosum

Renal
Proliferative glomerulonephritis (rare)

INVESTIGATIONS

FBC
Hb $\downarrow$ (MCV normal)
WCC $\uparrow$
Platelets $\uparrow$

U + Es
Normal

LFTs
Normal

ESR $\uparrow$
CRP $\uparrow$
Autoantibodies to type II collagen are sometimes
  detectable but are non-specific

ECG
Variable degree of heart block

Echocardiography
Valve regurgitation
Aortic root dilatation

Audiometry
Conductive deafness

Renal biopsy may confirm glomerulonephritis

DIAGNOSIS

This is largely a clinical one, but biopsy evidence of chondritis helps confirm the diagnosis.

Cartilage biopsy
Histology of affected cartilage shows reduced chondrocytes, reduced basophilic staining and an inflammatory infiltrate.

DIFFERENTIAL DIAGNOSIS

Infectious perichondritis – usually with
  Pseudomonas aeruginosa

Causes of a collapsed bridge of nose ('saddle nose')
Wegener's granulomatosis
Congenital syphilis
Trauma
Lepromatous leprosy
Sarcoid
Cutaneous leishmaniasis
Lupus vulgaris

Note that leprosy, sarcoid, leishmaniasis and TB have other changes seen in the skin.

TREATMENT

NSAIDs for pain

Steroids in high dose may help in acute disease, but disease progression may carry on regardless. Immunosuppression has been used with cyclosporin, azothioprine and cyclophosphamide.

Reconstruction of tracheal cartilage, and aortic valve replacement are sometimes required.

PROGNOSIS

25% 5 year mortality mostly due to tracheal collapse or cardiovascular complications.

QUESTION SPOTTING

Grey case

Consider relapsing polychondritis if conductive deafness and polyarthritis or cardiovascular complication, especially in the presence of a saddle nose.

Data interpretation

You may be asked to interpret an audiometry report in the context of symptoms or signs of polychondritis.

POLYMYOSITIS AND DERMATOMYOSITIS

Polymyositis is a connective tissue disease which causes inflammation and necrosis of muscle fibres. When accompanied by a rash it is known as dermatomyositis. It affects women more than men. It may run an acute course or a more chronic course.

There are five categories of disease:
1) Adult polymyositis
2) Adult dermatomyositis
3) Dermatomyositis or polymyositis with malignancy
4) Childhood dermatomyositis
5) Polymyositis as part of other connective tissue disease

CLINICAL FEATURES

Muscles
Proximal muscle weakness esp. affecting shoulder and pelvic girdles
Muscle tenderness or pain in approx 50%
Muscle wasting (occurs later than the weakness)

Pharyngeal and respiratory muscle involvement may cause dysphagia, dysphonia, and respiratory failure.

Skin
'Heliotrope' rash (25%)
Gottron's papules (violet, scaly rash on knuckles)
Rash on elbows, knees (30–50%)
Cutaneous and muscular calcification
Loss of skin elasticity may give appearances similar to systemic sclerosis

Nail fold changes
Periungual erythema
Cuticular hypertrophy
Infarcts

Cardiac
Often asymptomatic
Heart block
Arrhythmias
Myocardial infarction
Pericarditis

Other
Fever
Weight loss
Mild arthralgia or inflammatory polyarthritis affecting the small joints of the hands

Raynaud's syndrome in 30%
Renal involvement is rare except if myoglobinuria causes renal impairment
Pulmonary fibrosis (particularly associated with the Jo-1 antibody)

INVESTIGATIONS

FBC
Hb $\downarrow$ (MCV normal)
WCC $\uparrow$ if severe with neutrophilia
Platelets normal or $\uparrow$

U + Es
Na normal
K normal
Urea and creatinine $\uparrow$ if myoglobinuria causes renal impairment

LFTs
AST $\uparrow$
Albumin $\downarrow$
Otherwise normal

ESR $\uparrow$
Immunoglobulins may be $\uparrow$ especially IgG
ANA usually positive
Jo-1 positive 30% and is a marker for pulmonary fibrosis
Rheumatoid factor may be positive

In older patients a basic search for malignancy with chest X-ray, mammogram, tumour markers and maybe a pelvic ultrasound is recommended, although some advocate that this is not indicated unless there is clinical suspicion of malignancy.

DIAGNOSIS

CK $\uparrow$

EMG
Shows myopathy and denervation. The typical triad includes:

Short polyphasic motor units
Spontaneous fibrillation
High frequency repetitive discharges

Muscle biopsy
Muscle fibre necrosis and inflammation with regeneration, but may be normal as the inflammation can be patchy and may be missed by biopsy.

TREATMENT

Bed rest and limb splinting to prevent contractures.

High dose steroids.

CK falls before muscle strength returns. Monitor both while reducing steroid dose.

Physiotherapy once muscle strength begins to return.

Immunosuppression with azathioprine or methotrexate may be required if steroids fail.

PROGNOSIS

Poor in children who also suffer long-term morbidity if they survive.

Poor prognosis with cardiac involvement or pulmonary fibrosis.

DIFFERENTIAL DIAGNOSIS

Connective tissue disorders – SLE, scleroderma, MCTD, rheumatoid arthritis

Other vasculitides – polyarteritis nodosa, giant cell arteritis/polymyalgia rheumatica

Myasthenia gravis

Muscular dystrophy

Endocrine myopathy – thyrotoxicosis, hypothyroidism, osteomalacia

Drug induced myopathy

Infective myositis

Malignant myopathy

Neurogenic atrophy

QUESTION SPOTTING

Grey case

The difficulty will be in differentiating polymyositis with multisystem involvement from SLE or scleroderma. Polymyalgia can be differentiated by the muscle stiffness and the lack of wasting. Abnormal AST or CK in the absence of other abnormal LFTs point to a myositis. The pattern of the clinical disease should lead directly to the diagnosis.

Data interpretation

May require you to interpret the EMG findings.

FAMILIAL MEDITERRANEAN FEVER

FMF, or recurrent polyserositis, is an inflammatory disease characterized by recurrent episodes of neutrophilic inflammation of serosal and joint surfaces. A gene on chromosome 16 has now been cloned and is thought to underlie most cases of the disease; its exact role in regulation of the inflammatory response is unclear at present. FMF mostly affects patients from Greece, Turkey and North Africa. 80% present by the age of 20; 99% present by the age of 40.

Attacks build rapidly to a peak over a few hours, and resolve over the next few days.

SYMPTOMS

Abdominal pain; starting in one area, rapidly
  spreading
Fever
Vomiting
Constipation
Pleuritic chest pain (50%)
Joint pain and swelling (25–80%)

SIGNS

Fever
Tachycardia
Abdominal tenderness, with rebound and
  guarding
Reduced bowel sounds
Inflamed large joints
Splenomegaly (30%)

Other features

Headache
Skin rash: hot, red and tender, extensor surfaces
  (10–20%)
Small pleural effusion; pericarditis (less
  common), pleural rub is rare

INVESTIGATIONS

FBC
Hb slightly ↓
WCC ↑
Platelets usually normal

U + Es
Raised in amyloidosis

LFTs
Usually normal

ESR ↑
CRP ↑
Immunoglobulins ↑
Amylase normal
ANA negative
Rheumatoid factor negative

Urine
Blood
Protein if amyloidosis

DIAGNOSIS

Usually a diagnosis of exclusion. Family history and recovery from multiple bouts of acute abdominal pain associated with peritonitis are pointers. PCR to look for the FMF gene should give the diagnosis in future.

DIFFERENTIAL DIAGNOSIS

Any cause of acute abdomen
Septic arthritis
Juvenile RA
SLE
Rheumatic fever
AIP
Crohn's disease
Multiple pulmonary emboli

COMPLICATIONS

AA type amyloidosis occurs in 25%, with renal failure the usual end result.
  Amyloidosis can be prevented, and probably reversed once established, by colchicine.

TREATMENT

Colchicine prevents attacks in 95% of sufferers, and can prevent amyloidosis.

PROGNOSIS

Normal life expectancy in the absence of amyloidosis.

QUESTION SPOTTING

Grey case
Clues to a diagnosis of FMF are:
Family history of recurrent abdominal pain
Mediterranean origin
Peritonitis that improves on its own over a
  couple of days

Recurrent attacks of abdominal and joint pain
  plus fever
Negative ANA and rheumatoid factor

Data interpretation
The disease is much more likely to come up as a
grey case than as a data interpretation.

CHURG-STRAUSS SYNDROME

Churg-Strauss syndrome is a combination of granulomatous necrotizing vasculitis of small to medium sized vessels and eosinophilic pneumonia in association with asthma and peripheral eosinophilia. The disease tends to start with an allergic rhinitis with asthma. This usually develops into a blood, lung and gastrointestinal eosinophilia. The final stage is a systemic vasculitis when the asthma may recede. The syndrome is rare. There is slight male preponderance, and the mean age of onset is 40–50 years old.

CLINICAL FEATURES

General
Seen once systemic vasculitis occurs:
Fever
Weight loss
Fatigue
Myalgia
Arthralgia

Respiratory
Allergic rhinitis and eosinophilic sinusitis – usually the first feature, and seen in young adulthood
Nasal polyposis

Asthma – typically severe and adult in onset.

Nervous system (60%)
Mononeuritis multiplex
Polyneuropathy – distal and symmetrical or asymmetrical
Radiculopathies
Optic neuropathy

Cranial nerve lesions inc. trigeminal neuropathy.
    Central nervous manifestations such as psychiatric disturbance, stroke, epilepsy have all been reported but are rare.

Skin (60%)
Vasculitis rash – palpable purpura of the lower extremities.
    Subcutaneous granulomatous nodules.
    Livedo reticularis, bullous lesions, urticaria and maculopapular lesions all seen rarely.

Renal (20–50%)
Focal segmental glomerulonephritis occurs but less common and severe than polyarteritis nodosa.

Gastrointestinal system
Abdominal pain – indicates eosinophilic mass lesions which may cause obstruction or ulceration and haemorrhagic diarrhoea.
    Fistulae, perforation also seen.
    Pancreatitis.
    Acute acalculous cholecystitis.

Haematological
Peripheral eosinophilia
Autoimmune haemolytic anaemia (rare)

Cardiac
Myocardial infarction from coronary artery vasculitis
Heart failure from eosinophilic myocardial infiltration
Mitral regurgitation in the absence of heart failure, possibly due to myocardial fibrosis
Conduction defects

INVESTIGATIONS

FBC
Hb $\downarrow$ (normal MCV)
WCC $\uparrow$ or normal but eosinophils $\uparrow$ ($>1.5 \times 10^9$/l or >10% of differential)
Platelets normal

U + Es
Na and K normal
Urea and creatinine $\uparrow$ if renal involvement

LFTs
Albumin $\downarrow$
Otherwise normal

ESR $\uparrow$
CRP $\uparrow$
Immunoglobulins often $\uparrow$ with $\uparrow\uparrow$ IgE
ANCA positive in 60% (usually pANCA, but may be cANCA cf. Wegener's granulomatosis which tends to be cANCA positive and polyarteritis nodosa which is usually ANCA negative)
Rheumatoid factor may be positive or negative
ANA usually negative

Diagnosis may be made from the history, ESR ↑ and rapid response to steroids.

TREATMENT

Polymyalgia rheumatica

Steroids: prednisolone 10–20 mg/day for 1 month, then a reducing dose to maintenance of 5–7.5 mg/day. Steroids may be required for 3–4 years, but it is worth attempting withdrawal by 2 years.

Giant cell arteritis

Steroids: prednisolone 40 mg/day (80 mg if any ocular symptoms) for 2 months, then reduce dose. If dose reduction is difficult due to ongoing symptoms or persistently raised ESR, then azathioprine or methotrexate may be used as steroid sparing agents.

PROGNOSIS

Relapses are common and may occur in up to 30%. Giant cell arteritis may be fatal if basilar artery occlusion occurs.

DIFFERENTIAL DIAGNOSIS

Multiple myeloma
Rheumatoid arthritis
Connective tissue diseases
Polymyositis
Neoplasia with paraneoplastic syndrome

QUESTION SPOTTING

Grey case

The diagnosis is almost exclusive to the over 50 year old population. The typical patient will be a white, female 60–70 year old with non-specific aches and pains particularly in the morning. A history of headaches should give the diagnosis away. If the symptoms and ESR do not resolve rapidly with steroids consideration of alternative diagnoses such as malignancy is imperative.

Data interpretation

Less likely to appear in this section.

ENDOCRINE DISEASE

CUSHING'S SYNDROME

Chronic inappropriate hypersecretion of cortisol, as a result of several different disease processes:

1. High ACTH levels
Pituitary microadenoma (Cushing's disease)
Ectopic ACTH (e.g. small cell lung cancer)

2. Primary hypercortisolaemia
Adrenal hyperplasia
Adrenal tumour (carcinoma or adenoma)
Exogenous steroids

3. Ectopic CRF production (very rare)

SYMPTOMS

Weakness, especially proximal (30–50%)
Easy bruising (60%)
Reduced libido
Dysmenorrhoea (80%)
Depression, psychosis (60%)
Weight gain (>90%)

SIGNS

Moon face, buffalo hump (90%)
Centripetal obesity
Hirsutism (80%)
Red abdominal striae (50%)
Acne
Hyperpigmentation (if ACTH raised)
Ankle oedema (50%)
Hypertension (75%)
Proximal muscle weakness

Other features
Osteoporosis and fractures (20%)
Diabetes or impaired glucose tolerance (50%)
Renal calculi (15%)
Frequent infections

NB. Ectopic ACTH secretion by small cell lung cancer may produce a body habitus not dissimilar to Addison's disease, with weight loss and pigmentation.

INVESTIGATIONS

FBC
Usually normal

U + Es
Na normal
K may be very ↓ esp. if ectopic ACTH
Urea usually normal
Creatinine usually normal

LFTs
Normal

Calcium usually normal
Bicarbonate often elevated
Glucose often elevated

Chest X-ray can show evidence of small cell lung cancer

CT of adrenals may show adrenal adenoma or carcinoma. If pituitary or ectopic ACTH production, bilateral adrenal enlargement will be seen. Note 8% of population have 'incidentalomas'.

MRI pituitary can show pituitary microadenomas.

DIAGNOSIS

1) Is there hypercortisolism?
Midnight cortisol: Normal circadian rhythm is lost in Cushing's syndrome, thus 2400 h cortisol is greater than 180 nmol/L. Infection and the stress of recent hospital admission will also give high readings.

24 h urinary free cortisol: Elevated in 95% of Cushing's syndrome. False positive rate is 1–5%

Short dexamethasone suppression test: 2 mg dexamethasone taken between 2200 and 2400 hours. Plasma cortisol taken at 0900 to 1100 hours. Normal ″250 nmol/L

Low dose dexamethasone suppression test: 0.5 mg dexamethasone given 6 hourly for 48 h. Plasma cortisol then measured. Normal: < 50 nmol/L

2) What is the cause?
Plasma ACTH measurement. High levels suggest pituitary or ectopic ACTH secretion. Suppressed levels indicate adrenal source or exogenous steroid. Levels above 300 ng/L are usually due to ectopic ACTH secretion

High dose dexamethasone suppression test: Measure 0900 cortisol at start, then give 2 mg dexamethasone 6 hourly for 48 h. Suppression to less than 50% of basal level suggests pituitary origin for the high ACTH. Lack of suppression suggests an ectopic source.

Venous sampling from inferior petrosal sinuses: If ACTH concentration is much higher in the sinuses than in the peripheral circulation, a pituitary source of ACTH is probable.

DIFFERENTIAL DIAGNOSIS

Alcoholism – 'pseudo-Cushing's'
Severe intercurrent illness

Depression (can be very difficult to differentiate; depressed patients raise their cortisol in response to an insulin stress test; patients with Cushing's do not).

TREATMENT

Pituitary adenoma: Surgery plus radiotherapy. Successful in 75–80%.
Adrenal adenoma: Surgery.
Ectopic source: Surgery, radiotherapy or chemotherapy.

Metyrapone is useful prior to surgery, as it blocks cortisol production and thus allows control of BP, improves wound healing, stops weight gain and reduces the risk of infection. Ketoconazole is an alternative.

QUESTION SPOTTING

Grey case
Good discriminating features for Cushing's include:

Thin skin, easy bruising
Proximal myopathy
Facial plethora

Consider Cushing's if a hypokalaemic metabolic alkalosis is present.

Another classic presentation is the patient who is a smoker with weight loss, pigmentation, hypertension and a metabolic alkalosis – small cell lung cancer being the diagnosis.

Data interpretation
As above, but more commonly, you will be asked to interpret the results of a dexamethasone suppression test in one form or another.

ACROMEGALY

Excessive growth hormone secretion, usually from a pituitary adenoma (>95%). Symptoms are caused by mass effect from the adenoma as well as by the effects of growth hormone. 3% of patients with acromegaly have GHRH secretion from tumours in the hypothalamus, adrenal, pancreas or from carcinoid tumours. Less than 2% of cases are due to GH secreting islet cell tumours.

Overall, 6% of acromegalics have the MEN 1 syndrome.

SYMPTOMS

Mass effect
Headache
Visual impairment
Diplopia

Hormonal
Deepening of voice
Enlarging hands, feet, jaw
Sweating

Joint pains (60–70%)
Snoring
Impotence (25–45%)
Dysmenorrhoea (30–85%)
Weakness
Numbness, paraesthesia

SIGNS

Mass effect
Cranial nerve palsies (III, IV, VI)
Bitemporal hemianopia

Hormonal
Frontal bossing
Prognathism, malocclusion
'Spade like' hands
Thick, oily skin
Acanthosis nigricans
Carpal tunnel syndrome
Hypertension
Palpable thyroid
Palpable kidneys

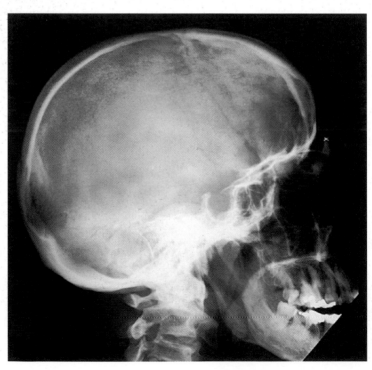

Fig. 10.   Acromegaly. A lateral skull X-ray showing enlarged pituitary fossa and enlarged jaw typical of acromegaly.

Cardiac enlargement
Large tongue

INVESTIGATIONS

FBC
Usually normal

U + Es
Usually normal

LFTs
Usually normal
Calcium normal

Glucose often ↑ (10–20% are diabetic, 30–45% have impaired glucose tolerance)

Cholesterol normal
Triglycerides ↑
IGF-1 ↑
Prolactin ↑ in 40%
LH, FSH may be ↓

Urinary calcium ↑

SXR
May show enlarged pituitary fossa (see Fig. 10)
Thickened skull
Enlarged frontal sinuses
Malocclusion

Foot XR may show thickened heel pad
Hand XR shows large phalanges, phalangeal tufts

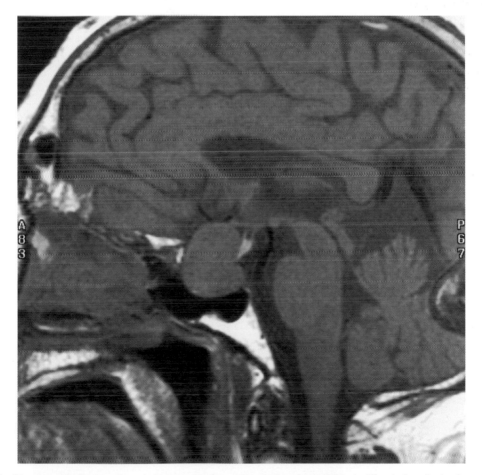

Fig. 11. Acromegaly. An enlarged pituitary gland on a T1 weight sagittal MRI brain. The pituitary is clearly enlarged and extends both superiorly and posteriorly from the pituitary fossa.

MRI brain often shows pituitary adenoma; most are macroadenomas (see Fig. 11)

DIAGNOSIS

IGF-1 levels almost always raised; low levels effectively rule out acromegaly.

Glucose Tolerance Test (GTT): 75 g glucose load is taken after fasting. In normal individuals, GH levels are suppressed to <2 mcg/L. The GTT may also show evidence of diabetes or impaired glucose tolerance.

MRI of the pituitary to detect the adenoma – see Fig. 11.

DIFFERENTIAL DIAGNOSIS

Acromegaly plus panhypopituitarism
Acromegaly as part of MEN 1
Haemochromatosis (Diabetes + joint pains)
Other pituitary adenomas (mass effects), especially prolactinoma

COMPLICATIONS

Glucose intolerance or diabetes
Obstructive sleep apnoea
Panhypopituitarism
Cardiomyopathy (20–40%)

TREATMENT

Transsphenoidal hypophysectomy: 60% success rate; 1–9% diabetes insipidus
Radiotherapy post surgery if control is inadequate (GH >5 mcg/L)

Bromocriptine, cabergoline, octreotide or lanreotide to control symptoms (successful in 70–90%) and as a holding measure. The dopamine antagonists bromocriptine and cabergoline are less effective than octreotide, and the long acting analogue lanreotide.

PROGNOSIS

Life expectancy is reduced in acromegaly, but there is no evidence (yet) that cure improves life expectancy.

QUESTION SPOTTING

Grey case

Perhaps less likely to occur as a grey case, as the full set of clinical features are quite distinctive. If it does occur, beware coexistent panhypopituitarism, or a cause other than a pituitary adenoma.

Data interpretation

Most likely to occur in the context of interpreting a glucose tolerance test.

ACUTE INTERMITTENT PORPHYRIA

An autosomal dominant condition caused by inheriting an inactive allele of porphobilinogen (PBG) deaminase. This leads to reduced PBG deaminase activity and build up of porphyrin precursors, particularly delta-aminolaevulinic acid. The features of the disease result from the neurotoxic effects of δ-ALA on motor, sensory, central and autonomic nerves.

Attacks occur intermittently, being precipitated by intercurrent infection, fasting, pregnancy, parturition and a variety of drugs, including alcohol.

SYMPTOMS

Abdominal pain (95%)
Vomiting
Constipation
Depression and anxiety, hallucinations and psychosis (50%)
Weakness, often starting peripherally. May progress to respiratory paralysis and difficulty swallowing
Paraesthesia
Convulsions

SIGNS

Tachycardia, hypertension, postural drop (70%)
Pyrexia
Sweating
Mild abdominal tenderness
Bowel sounds usually normal
Lower motor neurone weakness

INVESTIGATIONS

FBC
Hb normal
WCC $\uparrow$ (neutrophilia)
Platelets normal

U + Es
Na $\downarrow$ (due to SIADH)
K $\downarrow$
Urea $\uparrow$

LFTs
Often abnormal

Abdominal X-ray normal or shows colonic dilatation

Urine shows proteinuria. Urine darkens on standing.

DIAGNOSIS

Ehrlichs test: Add one volume Ehrlichs reagent to one volume of urine. Sample turns red. Add two volumes of chloroform. Red colour stays in upper (aqueous) layer in AIP.
Urinary δ-ALA and porphobilinogen both raised.
Erythrocyte PBG deaminase levels are decreased.

DIFFERENTIAL DIAGNOSIS

SLE
Acute lead poisoning
Drug intoxication
Toxaemia of pregnancy

COMPLICATIONS

Death can occur from respiratory paralysis or aspiration, and the autonomic instability is thought to be the underlying reason for sudden death in some cases.

Chronic abdominal pain, weakness and paraesthesia can occur as long-term neurological sequelae, and 40% of patients remain hypertensive between attacks.

TREATMENT

High carbohydrate intake
Morphine for analgesia
Fluid replacement
β blockade for tachycardia/hypertension

Chlorpromazine and a dark, quiet environment for psychosis and agitation.

Monitor for respiratory embarrassment (FVC)

There is some evidence that using IV Haem arginate reduces the duration and severity of attacks.

QUESTION SPOTTING

Grey case

May present as abdominal pain and constipation
but no tenderness

Past history of psychosis or fits

Pregnant or post-parturition women on diazepam
who present with collapse.

Data interpretation

AIP is less likely to come up as a data
interpretation question, but the key findings are:

Low sodium
Raised LFTs
Raised WCC

A possible differential here would include lead
poisoning, drug intoxication and atypical
pneumonias.

Abdominal pain + low sodium: Think of AIP.

ADDISON'S DISEASE

Addison's disease refers to primary failure of the adrenal cortex, with consequent loss of production of glucocorticoids and mineralocorticoids.

Causes

Autoimmune adrenalitis (70–80%) – antibodies can be found against the 21-hydroxylase enzyme in 90% of autoimmune cases.

Tuberculosis
Metastatic malignancy, especially small cell lung cancer and lymphoma
Amyloidosis
Haemorrhage/infarction
Bilateral adrenalectomy
AIDS – caused by infections, e.g. CMV, PCP, fungi
Adrenoleucodystrophy

SYMPTOMS

Tiredness
Depression
Anorexia
Weight loss
Nausea and vomiting
Abdominal pain
Diarrhoea
Dizziness
Myalgia
Amenorrhoea (uncommon)

SIGNS

Pigmentation (90%) on sun exposed areas, mucosal surfaces, axillae, palmar creases and in recent scars.

Loss of body hair
Cachexia
Postural hypotension (lying BP may be normal)
Low grade fever

Rare features

Benign intracranial hypertension
Proximal myopathy
Peripheral neuropathy

Addisonian crises

Characterized by dehydration and hypotension. Coma and fits may occur. Crises may be precipitated by surgery, trauma, infection or other major illness, particularly where gastrointestinal fluid loss is prominent.

INVESTIGATIONS

FBC

Hb may $\downarrow$ after rehydration
WCC normal or $\uparrow$ (may show eosinophilia or lymphocytosis)
Platelets normal

U + Es

Na $\downarrow$ in 90%
K $\uparrow$ in 65%
Urea often $\uparrow$
Creatinine may be $\uparrow$

LFTs

Usually normal
Calcium may rise after rehydration
HCO_3 may be $\downarrow$ in crisis
Glucose $\downarrow$ in 50%

TFTs may show $\uparrow$ TSH and $\downarrow$ T_4. May be due to coexistent hypothyroidism or may revert to normal with corticosteroids.

Adrenal antibodies: present in 90% of cases due to autoimmune adrenalitis. Rare in other causes of Addison's.

Chest X-ray may show evidence of lung cancer or TB.

Abdominal X-ray may show adrenal calcification from TB.

DIAGNOSIS

Short synacthen test. 250 mcg tetracosactrin given IM. Cortisol and ACTH taken at 0, 30 and 60 min. Plasma cortisol should rise by at least 250 ng/L compared with baseline, reaching >550 ng/L by 30 min.

Failure to achieve these levels suggests adrenal insufficiency. A high ACTH level is good evidence of primary adrenal failure.

Note also that renin levels are $\uparrow$, with normal or $\downarrow$ aldosterone.

Basal cortisol and urinary free cortisol are usually low normal and are thus much less useful in making the diagnosis.

ASSOCIATIONS

Autoimmune Addison's is associated with other autoimmune diseases sharing the HLA B8, DR3 haplotype, e.g.

IDDM
Pernicious anaemia
Thyroiditis/hypothyroidism
Vitiligo
Hypoparathyroidism
Primary ovarian failure

DIFFERENTIAL DIAGNOSIS

Beware syndromes which include Addison's disease, e.g. Schmidt's syndrome, polyglandular syndromes.

Panhypopituitarism
Diuretic use (especially potassium sparing
    diuretics)
Psychological
Chronic fatigue syndrome

TREATMENT

Addisonian crisis
IV normal saline 2–4 L over 24 h plus IV hydrocortisone 200–400 mg in 24 h. Correct hypoglycaemia with IV dextrose. Treat underlying infection or other precipitant of crisis.

Maintenance
Oral hydrocortisone, e.g. 20 mg morning, 10 mg evening. If postural hypotension or electrolyte abnormalities persist, fludrocortisone should be added in a dose of 50–200 mcg per day. A medic-alert bracelet, plus patient education to double the dose of steroid when unwell, are both essential.

QUESTION SPOTTING

Grey case
Key features are a non-specific history of
    tiredness, anorexia and GI symptoms
Dizziness with postural hypotension
Low sodium, with or without a high
    potassium

Data interpretation
May present as an abridged version of the above, or as the result of a short synacthen test to interpret.

HYPOPARATHYROIDISM

Underactivity of the parathyroid glands, or insensitivity to the effects of PTH (pseudohypoparathyroidism). Causes of hypoparathyroidism include:

Thyroid/parathyroid/neck surgery (>90%)
Familial
Sporadic (autoimmune)
DiGeorge syndrome
Hypomagnesaemia
Wilson's disease – rare
Haemochromatosis – rare
Metastatic malignancy – rare

SYMPTOMS

Paraesthesia
Abdominal pain
Muscle spasm and tetany
Emotional lability
Memory impairment
Seizures
Diarrhoea

SIGNS

Chvostek's sign (occurs in 5% of normal
    population)
Trousseau's sign
Dry skin
Grooved nails
Papilloedema
Cataracts

Somatic features associated with pseudohypoparathyroidism
Round face, short neck
Short stature
Short metacarpals and metatarsals, especially 4th
    and 5th
Osteitis fibrosa

INVESTIGATIONS

FBC
Normal

U + Es
Normal

LFTs
Normal (unless underlying liver disease)

Calcium $\downarrow$
PO_4 $\uparrow$

PTH $\downarrow$ or absent in hypoparathyroidism but $\uparrow$ in
    pseudohypoparathyroidism
CK may be $\uparrow$
Calcitriol $\downarrow$

Urine shows $\downarrow$ phosphate
ECG may show long QT interval

Hand XR shows short metacarpals
    (pseudohypoparathyroidism)
CT brain shows calcification of basal ganglia;
    other areas may also be affected

DIAGNOSIS

Low calcium plus raised phosphate in the
absence of other causes, e.g. renal failure,
malabsorption, osteomalacia.
    Chase-Auerbach test: Infusion of PTH,
causing:

$\uparrow$ urinary cAMP and PO_4 in hypoparathyroidism
No rise in urinary cAMP or PO_4 in complete
    pseudohypoparathyroidism
$\uparrow$ in urinary cAMP only in partial
    pseudohypoparathyroidism

ASSOCIATIONS

Hypothyroidism
Diabetes mellitus
Gonadal dysgenesis
Dysmenorrhoea
Blue sclerae (uncommon)

Autoimmune hypoparathyroidism is associated with:
Pernicious anaemia
Addison's disease
Polyglandular endocrine syndromes

NB. Somatic features of
    pseudohypoparathyroidism without
    hypocalcaemia constitute a partially expressed
    disease phenotype;
    pseudopseudohypoparathyroidism

TREATMENT

Calcium plus calcitriol or 1-alpha calcidol

PROGNOSIS

Good, but cataracts may not be prevented by
   normalizing calcium

QUESTION SPOTTING

Grey case

Perhaps less likely in this section, but look out
for the typical body habitus of
pseudohypoparathyroidism. Remember to look
for other features of APS-1 if
hypoparathyroidism is the diagnosis.

Data interpretation

Low calcium and high phosphate with normal
renal function and no evidence of malabsorption
point to the diagnosis.

Calcified basal ganglia or cataracts should
also alert you to the possibility of
hypocalcaemia.

MULTIPLE ENDOCRINE NEOPLASIA

MEN syndromes come in at least two types: MEN 1 is caused by a mutation on chromosome 11, MEN 2 by a mutation on chromosome 10 (the RET oncogene). Both types display autosomal dominant inheritance. MEN 2 is further divided into types a and b, based on the presence or absence of Marfanoid features.

MEN 1 CLINICAL FEATURES

Parathyroid hyperplasia (almost 100%)
Symptoms due to hypercalcaemia

Pancreatic endocrine tumours (40–70%)
Gastrinoma (60%): peptic ulcers, indigestion, diarrhoea
Insulinoma (30%)
Glucagonoma
VIPoma
Non-functioning adenomas

Pituitary adenomas (30–50%)
Prolactinoma (65%)
GH secreting (30%)
Others are rare

Carcinoid (5–10%)
Adrenal tumours (5–40%): usually non-functioning
Adrenal cortical hyperplasia
Lipomas (1%)

MEN 2 CLINICAL FEATURES

Medullary C cell thyroid carcinoma (MTC) (100%).
Phaeochromocytoma (50%) Bilateral in 70%.
2a: Parathyroid hyperplasia in 80%; often asymptomatic.
2b: Mucosal neuromas, marfanoid habitus, bowel neuromas – dysphagia, vomiting, megacolon, change in bowel habit. Parathyroid hyperplasia is rare.

INVESTIGATIONS

MEN 1
FBC
Normal

U + Es
Normal

LFTs
Usually normal
Calcium often raised
PO_4 often low

PTH often raised
Glucose normal, low or high (depending on pancreatic tumour)
Fasting gastrin raised in gastrinoma
Prolactin raised in prolactinoma
Insulin + C-peptide raised in insulinoma
Growth hormone, IGF-1 raised in acromegaly

MEN 2

FBC
Usually normal

U + Es
Usually normal

LFT
Usually normal

Calcitonin raised in MTC
Urinary catecholamines raised in phaeochromocytoma

DIAGNOSIS

Essentially clinical diagnosis based on two lesions occurring in a patient, or one characteristic lesion in a first degree relative of someone known to have the condition.
  Pentagastrin stimulation test is used to look for the presence of MTC; raised calcitonin levels following the test suggest the presence of MTC.

DIFFERENTIAL DIAGNOSIS

Other multiple neoplasia syndromes, e.g.
Von Hippel-Lindau syndrome
Neurofibromatosis
Mixed MEN (phaeochromocytoma + prolactinoma)
Hereditary MTC or phaeochromocytoma

TREATMENT

MEN 1
Treatment is that of the individual tumours. First and second degree relatives should be screened every 6 to 12 months with a history, examination,

calcium and prolactin levels, along with any tests for pancreatic or pituitary tumours suggested by the history and examination.

Genetic analysis can also now be used to identify those with the defective gene.

MEN 2

Again, the treatment is of the individual tumours, except for thyroid disease (see below).

Relatives of an index case should be genetically tested, and if positive, should undergo screening, as should anyone with a tumour associated with MEN 2 or any of the somatic features of the disease.

Screening should occur every 3 to 6 months in known cases and 6 to 12 monthly for carriers. History, examination, pentagastrin stimulation test, urinary catecholamines, PTH and calcium should be tested.

To reduce the risk of MTC, thyroidectomy can be done when the pentagastrin test is first abnormal, or at age 5 (MEN 2a) or age 2–3 (MEN 2b) – these are the earliest recorded ages of tumour occurrence.

QUESTION SPOTTING

Grey case

Consider MEN in anyone with:

Hyperparathyroidism
Unusual pancreatic tumour
Phaeochromocytomas
Multiple lipomas
Carcinoid

Also consider if a patient with a pituitary tumour presents with a second tumour.

Data interpretation

Less likely to occur, but a pentagastrin stimulation test result is possible.

AUTOIMMUNE POLYGLANDULAR SYNDROMES

Three types are recognised.

APS 1

Caused by a mutation in the APECED gene (chromosome 21). Defined as two of:

Addison's disease
Hypoparathyroidism
Chronic mucocutaneous candidiasis

Ectodermal dystrophy is a characteristic feature, and the onset is usually in childhood.

APS 2

Polygenic inheritance, with linkage to HLA DR3 and DR4. Adult onset. Defined as:

Addison's disease
plus either
Autoimmune thyroid disease or Type 1 diabetes mellitus

Schmidt's syndrome (Addison's + hypothyroidism) therefore falls within the definition of APS 2.

APS 3

Similar HLA linkage to APS 2. Defined as autoimmune thyroid disease plus at least one other autoimmune disorder in the absence of Addison's disease.

FEATURES OF SYNDROMES

APS 1

Autoimmune features
Hypoparathyroidism 80%
Ovarian failure 60%
Alopecia 30%
Malabsorption 20%
Testicular failure 15%
Pernicious anaemia 15%
Vitiligo 15%
Addison's disease 10%
IDDM 10%
Autoimmune hepatitis 10%
Hypothyroidism 5%

Ectodermal features
Candidiasis >95%
Enamel hypoplasia 80%
Nail dystrophy 50%
Keratopathy 35%
Tympanic membrane calcification 35%

Other associated manifestations reported include Sjögren's syndrome, asplenia, Turner's syndrome, vasculitis, hypophysitis and cholelithiasis.

APS 2

Addison's disease 100%
Thyroid disease 70%
IDDM 50%
Vitiligo 5%
Gonadal failure 5%
Hypopituitarism <1%
Alopecia <1%
Pernicious anaemia <1%
Candidiasis and hypoparathyroidism do not occur

INVESTIGATIONS

Results depend on which disease manifestations are present.
Addison's: $\uparrow$ K, $\downarrow$ Na, may have $\downarrow$ glucose and $\uparrow$ calcium. Urea $\uparrow$ if dehydrated.
Hypoparathyroidism: $\downarrow$ calcium, $\uparrow$ PO$_4$, $\downarrow$ PTH.
IDDM: $\uparrow$ glucose.
Pernicious anaemia: $\downarrow$ Hb, $\uparrow$ MCV, $\downarrow$ B$_{12}$. WCC and platelets may be $\downarrow$.
Thyroid disease: hyperthyroid or hypothyroid pattern of TFTs.
Hepatitis: abnormal LFTs, especially $\uparrow$ ALT.
Autoantibodies to the affected organs are usually present.

TREATMENT

Ketoconazole for candidiasis.
Autoimmune syndromes are treated in the same way as isolated disease would be treated.
Monitoring for the onset of associated disease manifestations is necessary.

PROGNOSIS

Good with treatment; probably 90% survival at 20 years from diagnosis.

QUESTION SPOTTING

Grey case

Any patient with candidal infection or hypoparathyroidism should raise the suspicion of APS 1.

For APS 2, cases of hypothyroidism that have extra features (e.g. a postural BP drop) should prompt consideration of APS 2.

Data interpretation

Less likely to crop up, but the above applies.

HYPOPITUITARISM

Hypopituitarism is the partial or complete loss of anterior pituitary hormone secretion as a result of either pituitary or hypothalamic disease.

Causes

Congenital
Familial hypopituitarism – very rare inherited disorder
Isolated hormone deficiencies, e.g. Kallman's syndrome (isolated GnRH deficiency)

Neoplastic
Pituitary adenomas
Para-pituitary tumours – meningiomas, gliomas, metastases, craniopharyngiomas

Vascular
Pituitary apoplexy
Sheehan's syndrome
Carotid artery aneurysm

Infective
Tuberculosis
Syphilis
Fungal
Abscesses

Trauma
Basal skull fracture
Pituitary surgery

Infiltrative
Haemochromatosis
Sarcoidosis
Wegener's granulomatosis

Other
Pituitary irradiation
Empty sella syndrome
Chemotherapy

The most common causes are pituitary tumours. Microadenomas rarely cause hypopituitarism, but with progressive enlargement of a pituitary adenoma, there is a sequential loss of pituitary function often in the context of excess secretion from the adenoma itself. In general, growth hormone (GH) is lost first, followed by luteinizing hormone (LH) and follicle stimulating hormone (FSH). Adrenocorticotrophic hormone (ACTH) is lost later and finally thyroid stimulating hormone (TSH).

CLINICAL FEATURES

This largely depends on the underlying cause and the hormonal axis lost. Below are the features expected for each deficiency.

Growth hormone deficiency

Children
Growth retardation

Adults
Reduced strength
Reduced muscle mass
Central obesity
Fatigue
Premature atherosclerosis

Gonadotropin deficiency

Men
Reduced libido
Erectile dysfunction
Impaired fertility
Loss of facial and body hair
Fine facial wrinkles
Gynaecomastia
Loss of bone mass
Loss of muscle mass and strength

Women
Altered menstrual function ranging from anovulatory regular cycles through to amenorrhoea.
Hot flushes.
Reduced libido.
Vaginal dryness with dyspareunia.
Pubic and axillary hair is preserved unless there is also loss of ACTH.

Post-menopausal women tend to present with either symptoms of the cause, e.g. headaches with visual field loss, or symptoms of other hormone deficiencies.

Corticotrophin deficiency
Fatigue
Weakness
Headache
Dizziness
Anorexia
Nausea, vomiting
Abdominal pain
Altered mental activity

Loss of axillary and pubic hair

Pallor

Hypoglycaemia

Anaemia (MCV normal) with eosinophilia may be seen.

Note that there is no hyperpigmentation as seen in primary adrenal failure, and that the typical findings of profound $\downarrow$ Na and $\uparrow$ K which are due to loss of aldosterone production in primary adrenal failure do not tend to be seen in hypopituitarism. Mild $\downarrow$ Na can occur due to $\uparrow$ vasopressin production.

Thyrotrophin deficiency

Symptoms

Fatigue

Weakness

Weight gain

Puffiness

Constipation

Cold intolerance

Children may be growth retarded, and with severe hypothyroidism, impairment of memory and mental activity can be noted

Signs

Bradycardia

Periorbital oedema

Slow relaxing reflexes

Prolactin deficiency or excess

Prolactin production is inhibited under normal circumstances, and loss does not usually cause any problems. However, hyperprolactinoma is more common.

This may either be due to a prolactin secreting macroadenoma or due to loss of inhibition by dopamine leading to increased prolactin production. A raised prolactin concentration is a good marker of pituitary dysfunction and may not necessarily indicate a prolactin secreting adenoma unless the levels are very high.

Hyperprolactinaemia

Galactorrhoea

Menstrual dysfunction, especially secondary amenorrhoea

INVESTIGATIONS

FBC

Hb $\downarrow$ or normal (MCV normal or $\uparrow$ If hypothyroid)

WCC normal

Platelets normal

U + Es

Na normal or $\downarrow$ if ACTH or TSH deficient

K usually normal

Urea and creatinine normal

LFTs

AST may be $\uparrow$ if thyroxine deficient

Otherwise normal

Creatinine kinase may be $\uparrow$ with thyroxine deficiency

DIAGNOSIS

Hormone testing (clearly depends on which hormones affected)

ACTH $\downarrow$

TSH – often in the normal range despite low T_4

Prolactin – may be $\uparrow$ or $\downarrow$ as noted above.

Thyroxine (T_4) $\downarrow$

Cortisol $\downarrow$

Oestradiol $\downarrow$

Testosterone $\downarrow$

LH $\downarrow$

FSH $\downarrow$

Dynamic testing (usually only required if partial loss of hormone makes diagnosis difficult)

Insulin stress test or glucagon stimulation test for growth hormone deficiency

Clomiphene test for gonadal function

Synacthen test for adrenal function

Imaging of pituitary fossa with MRI

DIFFERENTIAL DIAGNOSIS

Schmidt's syndrome

Addison's disease

Hypothyroidism

TREATMENT

Replacement of hormone deficiencies

Treatment of underlying condition if possible

Points to note:

Do not replace thyroxine until hypoadrenalism is excluded or treated as thyroxine may exacerbate cortisol deficiency.

Cortisol treatment may unmask a cranial diabetes insipidus, and this should be actively looked for after treatment commenced.

Cortisol replacement should be increased in times of stress such as surgery or infection.

Growth hormone has complicated interactions. Deficiency may make requirements of gonadotrophins higher for successful fertility in women and possibly men. Growth hormone replacement causes more conversion of T_4 to T_3 but this has no clinical significance. Growth hormone replacement may also reduce the availability of hydrocortisone, and may optimize glucose metabolism even if adequately replaced with cortisol, thyroxine and sex steroids.

QUESTION SPOTTING

Grey case

Hypopituitarism makes a good long case question. Some of the features are highly non-specific which can make diagnosis more difficult. The question should include a clue to the cause, such as previous trauma, headache or neurological disturbance.

Consider this diagnosis if the patient is pale in the absence of anaemia or if there is a history of reduced libido, amenorrhoea, or lethargy.

Data interpretation

Interpretation of hormone tests make hypopituitarism easy to put in this section. You may well be asked to work out which hormonal systems are affected.

OSTEOMALACIA

Lack of effect of vitamin D, either because of vitamin D deficiency, failure to convert precursors into the active vitamin, or resistance to the effects of vitamin D. Osteomalacia is the result in adults; rickets the result in children. The end result is defective mineralization of osteoid.

Causes of osteomalacia
Dietary lack
Lack of exposure to sunlight
Chronic renal failure
Liver failure
Anticonvulsants (esp. phenytoin, primidone, carbamazepine)

Malabsorption
Partial gastrectomy
Small bowel pathology
Biliary pathology

Inherited
Vitamin D resistant rickets
Fanconi's syndrome
Distal renal tubular acidosis
Vitamin D dependent rickets

Other
Phosphate binders
Laxatives
Bisphosphonates
Hyperparathyroidism
Hypoparathyroidism
Paraneoplastic

NB. Vitamin D resistant rickets is an X-linked condition where the renal tubule is insensitive to vitamin D. High urinary PO_4, low serum PO_4 but normal calcium and ALP result. Bone pain and weakness are uncommon, but the typical deformities of rickets occur, including short stature.

Vitamin D dependent rickets is a rare inherited disease of two types:
1) Low levels of 1,25 OH D, but normal levels of 25 OH D. This block in conversion can be overcome by giving more 25 OH D.
2) High levels of 1,25 OH D, but end-organ resistance. More 1,25 OH D is given.

SYMPTOMS

Bone pain, tenderness
Bone deformity
Weakness

SIGNS

Bony tenderness, pathological fractures
Proximal muscle weakness
Skeletal deformity (children), e.g. tibial bowing, rickety rosary, craniotabes, 'windswept' legs
Tetany (uncommon)
Enthesopathy; may lead to kyphosis and occasionally cord compression if gross deformity results

INVESTIGATIONS

FBC
Hb may be $\downarrow$ in GI tract disease
WCC usually normal
Platelets usually normal

U + Es
$\uparrow$ urea and creatinine in chronic renal failure

LFTs
ALP $\uparrow$
Calcium $\downarrow$ or low normal
$PO_4 \downarrow$

$HCO_3 \downarrow$
PTH $\uparrow$
Vitamin D $\downarrow$ in most cases

X-rays
Splayed metaphyses in children
Ragged appearance to growth plates
Looser's zones: commonest along femur, pubic bones, ribs, scapulae
Codfish (biconcave) vertebrae
Subperiosteal erosions on radial border of middle phalanges, resorption of clavicle ends and phalangeal tufts (due to secondary hyperparathyroidism)

DIAGNOSIS

Diagnosis can be confirmed by finding a low serum vitamin D level. Bone biopsy shows increased unmineralized osteoid.

Bone scan may show multiple undiagnosed pathological fractures.

DIFFERENTIAL DIAGNOSIS

For weakness and pains:

Polymyalgia rheumatica
Thyrotoxicosis
Cushing's syndrome
Polymyositis
Myeloma
Psychiatric pathology

TREATMENT

Replacement of vitamin D; usually precursor vitamin, but alfacalcidol or calcitriol in renal disease.

Phosphate supplements may be needed in vitamin D resistant rickets

QUESTION SPOTTING

Grey case

Clues to the diagnosis are:

Elderly, housebound patients or Asian women
Anyone on anticonvulsants
Anyone with GI tract disease
Vague aching symptoms
Diffuse weakness
Low calcium with elevated ALP

The important point with osteomalacia is not to stop once you have diagnosed the condition, but to go on and look for an underlying cause.

Data interpretation

Urinary calcium, phosphate and vitamin D metabolite levels may be given for interpretation.

HYPERPARATHYROIDISM

Inappropriately high levels of circulating parathyroid hormone (PTH). There are several causes.

Primary
Single adenoma (83%)
Parathyroid hyperplasia (11%)
Multiple adenomas (4%)
Parathyroid carcinoma (2%)

Secondary
Due to low calcium levels, e.g. renal failure, low vitamin D levels

Tertiary
Hyperfunction in the setting of secondary hyperparathyroidism

Ectopic
Due to release of PTH related peptide (PTHrP) from tumours, e.g. cancer of the lung. These peptides do not cross react with the normal PTH assay.

The following comments apply mainly to primary hyperparathyroidism.

Almost all features are due to hypercalcaemia.

SYMPTOMS

Usually asymptomatic (>70%)
Loin pain
Bone pain
Nausea
Vomiting
Polyuria, thirst
Arthritis
Mood swings, depression
Dementia, psychosis (uncommon)

SIGNS

Muscle hypotonicity
Band keratopathy
Hypertension (uncommon)
Proximal myopathy (uncommon)

OTHER FEATURES

Pseudogout
Nephrocalcinosis leading to renal failure
Peptic ulceration
Acute and chronic pancreatitis
Osteoporosis, fractures

INVESTIGATIONS

FBC
Normal

U + Es
Normal (unless chronic renal failure from nephrocalcinosis or dehydration)

LFTs
Bilirubin normal
ALT normal
ALP ↑ in 50%
Calcium ↑ (but may rarely be within normal range)
Phosphate ↓
ESR often ↑
PTH ↑ or inappropriately ↑ within normal range
Vitamin D usually normal
Chloride ↑
HCO_3 ↓
Mg often ↓

Immunoglobulins may show monoclonal band (even when no myeloma is present)

Urine
Calcium ↓
PO_4 ↑

ECG may show shortened QT interval

X-rays
Osteoporosis (especially at wrist)
Brown tumours (cysts)
Subperiosteal erosions, especially on radial border of middle phalanges
'Salt and pepper' skull and loss of lamina dura
Resorption of phalangeal tufts
Nephrocalcinosis on abdominal X-rays

DIAGNOSIS

1) Elevated calcium
2) Inappropriately raised PTH in presence of elevated calcium

Note that the PTH sample should be contemporaneous with the elevated calcium level. If measures to lower calcium are undertaken, the falling calcium level will trigger PTH release, even in situations (e.g. malignancy) where the PTH was previously suppressed. Thus hyperparathyroidism will be wrongly diagnosed.

DIFFERENTIAL DIAGNOSIS OF HYPERCALCAEMIA

High PTH
Primary or tertiary hyperparathyroidism

Low PTH
Malignancy (lung, breast, kidney, ovary, nasopharynx, myeloma, lymphoma, oesophagus)
Granulomas (sarcoid, TB, leprosy, histoplasmosis)
Drugs (lithium, vitamin A, vitamin D, milk alkali, oestrogens, thiazides)
Endocrine (thyrotoxicosis, phaeochromocytoma, VIPoma, Addisonian crisis)

Also beware a low albumin level (calcium needs correction), and prolonged cuffing prior to blood collection.

Familial hypocalciuric hypercalcaemia may also mimic hyperparathyroidism, with an inappropriately raised PTH. There are no symptoms however, and urinary calcium is low.

TREATMENT

Surgery if any of the following:

Ca >3.0
Osteopenia >2 SD below normal on DEXA scan
Age <50
Reduced creatinine clearance
Symptomatic disease
Urinary calcium >9 mmol/24 h

Otherwise, the disease may be observed.

Clodronate has been used in those not fit for surgery, but is unsuitable for long-term use

QUESTION SPOTTING

Grey case
The old saying 'Bones, stones, abdominal groans and psychic moans' is still relevant, but most cases are now picked up on routine blood testing, and are often asymptomatic elderly women.

Look for evidence of MEN if you suspect hyperparathyroidism

Data interpretation
If a high calcium plus raised PTH occurs, check that:
a) Specimen is uncuffed
b) Calcium is corrected
c) PTH was taken at same time as calcium, and calcium level was not falling
d) Urinary calcium is also raised before diagnosing primary hyperparathyroidism

CARCINOID SYNDROME

Episodic release of 5HT and other neuroendocrine mediators from tumours. The tumours are derived from neural crest cells, and often follow an indolent clinical course. They are usually found in the GI tract (90%) or in the lung (10%). Gut tumours cannot usually cause the carcinoid syndrome unless they have metastasized to the liver, as the liver is able to metabolize vasoactive mediators released into the portal vein by gut tumours. As a result, only 5–10% of carcinoid tumours produce the carcinoid syndrome.

Diversion of tryptophan away from niacin production into producing 5HT can lead to pellagra in chronic cases.

SYMPTOMS OF AN ATTACK

Flushing precipitated by alcohol
Wheezing
Dizziness

Other symptoms
Diarrhoea
Nausea, vomiting
Abdominal pain, especially RUQ pain
Dermatitis

SIGNS OF AN ATTACK

Tachycardia
Hypotension
Facial oedema

Other signs
Telangiectasia
Red/blue discoloration of face
RUQ tenderness, hepatomegaly (from metastases)
Dermatitis (from pellagra)
Depression, psychosis, tremor (from pellagra)
Abdominal mass (unusual)
Tricuspid regurgitation and/or pulmonary stenosis (50% of those with syndrome)
RV failure

NB. Bronchial carcinoids give rise to left-sided valve lesions

Other features
Arthritis
Sclerotic bone metastases

INVESTIGATIONS

FBC
Usually normal unless GI bleeding

U + Es
Usually normal

LFTs
May all be raised (metastases)

Echocardiography may demonstrate valvular lesions
U/S or CT abdomen may demonstrate liver metastases
CT thorax useful if symptomatic but no liver involvement; may show bronchial carcinoid

^{123}I-MIBG tracer scan: can show presence of metastases anywhere in the body

DIAGNOSIS

24 h urine collection showing raised levels of 5-HIAA. Need to avoid certain fruits prior to collection.

ASSOCIATIONS

Cushing's syndrome (some tumours also secrete ACTH)
MEN type 1

DIFFERENTIAL DIAGNOSIS

Anxiety attacks
Perimenopausal symptoms
Paroxysmal tachycardia
Phaeochromocytoma

TREATMENT

Surgery or embolization to bronchial tumours or solitary liver metastases
Octreotide improves symptoms in 90%
Nicotinamide to prevent pellagra
Radiotherapy may help pain from bone metastases

PROGNOSIS

5 year median survival; some patients may survive for up to 20 years

QUESTION SPOTTING

Grey case

Suspect carcinoid with:

Any right-sided heart lesion
Flushing episodes with low BP (cf. phaeochromocytoma)

Data interpretation

Less likely to occur in this section but may present as cardiac catheter data showing pulmonary stenosis.

NEUROLOGICAL DISEASE

7

SUBDURAL HAEMATOMA

Tearing of the veins in the arachnoid space, leading to accumulation of blood in the subdural space. Trauma is often mild, and is not recalled in 50% of patients with chronic subdural. The elderly, alcoholics, epileptics and those with cognitive impairment are especially at risk. Those taking anticoagulants are also at increased risk.

SYMPTOMS

Headache (25%)
Vomiting (10%)
Drowsiness
Limb weakness
Mood or personality change
Incontinence

SIGNS

Limb weakness / posturing (50%)
Dysphasia (20%)
Unequal pupils (15%)
Cranial nerve palsies (10–15%)
Fits (5–10%)
Extensor plantars (uncommon)

INVESTIGATIONS

FBC
Usually normal

U + Es
Usually normal

LFTs
Deranged in alcoholics

INR raised if on anticoagulants or alcoholic
SXR may show skull fracture

CT brain shows bright crescent if haematoma; appears isodense with brain after 1–2 weeks.

DIAGNOSIS

Made on CT scan result.

DIFFERENTIAL DIAGNOSIS

Intracranial tumour
Thromboembolic CVA
Subarachnoid haemorrhage
Extradural haematoma
Metabolic derangement (renal failure, liver failure, infection)
Cerebral abscess

TREATMENT

Surgical evacuation of haematoma
Small haematomas may resolve spontaneously

PROGNOSIS

Moderate to good outcome in 90%
Worse outcome with lower GCS

QUESTION SPOTTING

Grey case
Consider in any patient with neurological signs or reduced GCS, especially if:

They are on warfarin
They are elderly
There is a history of falls
They are alcoholic

Data interpretation
Unlikely to feature in this section.

NEUROFIBROMATOSIS

Loss of function by mutations in one of the two NF tumour suppressor genes. The disease is inherited in an autosomal dominant manner, but is expressed in different ways in different individuals – a wide variety of gene mutations has been described.

FEATURES (TYPE 1)

Diagnostic
a) Café au lait spots (>5, bigger than 15 mm in adults)
b) Lisch nodules in iris
c) Axillary freckling
d) Cutaneous neurofibromas, plexiform neurofibromas
e) Bone deformity and fractures, pseudoarthrosis
f) Optic glioma

Body habitus
Relative macrocephaly
Relative short stature
Kyphoscoliosis
Limb gigantism

Other neoplasms
Phaeochromocytoma
Neurofibromas of the spine, nerve roots and cranial nerves
Juvenile CML
Rhabdomyosarcoma
Wilm's tumour

Other neurological manifestations
May have reduced higher cerebral function (up to 40%)
Glaucoma
Migrainous headaches

Other systems
Arterial aneurysms
Renal artery stenosis: hypertension
GI bleeding, GI obstruction (neurofibromas)
Pulmonary fibrosis

FEATURES (TYPE 2)

Bilateral acoustic neuromas
Meningiomas
Schwannomas: cranial nerve, spinal, paraspinal

Gliomas, e.g. brainstem, cerebellum
Posterior lens opacification
Skin lesions (schwannomas or neurofibromas)
Retinal hamartomas

INVESTIGATIONS

FBC
Usually normal

U + Es
Usually normal

LFTs
Usually normal

CXR may show rib notching, normal or large lung fields. Neurofibromas may be visible.
MRI may reveal intracranial tumours, spinal tumours, and multiple high signal areas (NF-1) of unknown aetiology.
PFTs show normal FEV1 and FVC with reduced TLco.

DIAGNOSIS

For NF-1:
Two of: a) to f) or one plus an affected first degree relative.
For NF-2:
Bilateral acoustic neuroma

or

Affected first degree relative plus one of:
Unilateral acoustic neuroma by age 30
Meningioma
Glioma
Schwannoma
Posterior lens opacity in childhood

DIFFERENTIAL DIAGNOSIS

This depends on the context of the question. Possibilities are:

MEN 2 (for phaeochromocytoma)
Noonan's syndrome

For normal lung volumes with reduced TLco, consider:

Tuberose sclerosis

Lymphangioleiomyomatosis
Histiocytosis X

COMPLICATIONS

Plexiform neurofibromas may transform into sarcomatous lesions.
Cutaneous neurofibromas almost never do.
Renal artery stenosis and phaeochromocytoma may lead to hypertension.
Most complications are due to mass effects from tumours, and skeletal malformation / fracture.

TREATMENT

No treatment is curative; treatment is directed against specific lesions as they arise.

PROGNOSIS

Reduced life expectancy due to occurrence of tumours.

QUESTION SPOTTING

Grey case

Any previous neurological tumour should raise suspicion of neurofibromatosis, especially the presence of an acoustic neuroma.
Also consider the diagnosis in a patient with what sounds like a phaeochromocytoma.

Data interpretation

Less likely in this section, but remember the disease as a cause of large lungs with a reduced transfer factor.

BENIGN INTRACRANIAL HYPERTENSION (Pseudotumour cerebri)

Raised intracranial pressure in the absence of an intracranial mass lesion, and no enlargement of the ventricles due to hydrocephalus. The CSF composition is normal. The cause is unknown in most cases, but is important to exclude sagittal sinus thrombosis which may be associated with:

SLE
Pregnancy
Oral contraceptive pill
Essential thrombocythemia
Protein S deficiency
Antithrombin III deficiency
Antiphospholipid syndrome
Paroxysmal nocturnal haemoglobinuria
Behçet's disease
Meningeal sarcoidosis
Mastoiditis

However, other drugs and conditions may predispose to benign intracranial hypertension per se, without obstruction to venous outflow. These include:

Hypovitaminosis A
Hypervitaminosis A
Empty sella syndrome
Drugs such as nalidixic acid, nitrofurantoin, corticosteroids and tetracyclines

A likely mechanism of disease is a reduction in the reabsorption of CSF by the arachnoid villi although proof for this is lacking.

Benign intracranial hypertension is a rare disorder that is more common in women (over 90% being overweight) and particularly affects those between 18 and 40 years old.

SYMPTOMS

Headache
Throbbing
Worse on waking, straining, coughing and sneezing.

Visual disturbances
Transient and permanent visual loss
Photopsia – flashing lights
Blurring
Scotomata – enlarged blind spots are common

Diplopia due to 6th cranial nerve palsy (false localizing sign)
Colour vision is affected early in the disease

Pulsatile tinnitus
Retrobulbar pain

Note that cognitive function is preserved and seizures are rare, unlike mass lesions, hydrocephalus and viral and bacterial meningo-encephalopathy.

SIGNS

Papilloedema is almost always present – may be unilateral.

INVESTIGATIONS

FBC
Normal

U + Es
Normal

Other blood tests normal

Visual field analysis with formal perimetry – to look for blind spot enlargement, and scotomas. Most common are arcuate defects, nasal steps and global constriction of the visual fields.

Skull radiography is usually normal.

DIAGNOSIS

Lumbar puncture

Typically normal CSF composition, but with CSF pressure of >20 cm H_2O. However, the opening pressure may be normal, but a continuous pressure study may show pressure spikes.

CT head

Shows normal or slit like ventricles. Dural sinus thrombosis may be evident.

MR angiography
Sensitive for showing sinus thrombosis

DIFFERENTIAL DIAGNOSIS

Intracranial tumour
Sagittal sinus thrombosis
Subdural haematoma
Hydrocephalus
Sleep apnoea

TREATMENT

Aims to alleviate symptoms and preserve
  sight
Weight reduction – now of proven value
Carbonic anhydrase inhibitors, e.g.
  acetazolamide
Loop diuretics
Corticosteroids – beware of the complications
  in this group of already overweight
  patients
Repeat lumbar puncture – no proven benefit as
  the CSF pressure only remains low for about
  1–2 h after the puncture, but is still used on
  occasion

Surgical treatments
Lumboperitoneal shunt
Effective but complications of general
  anaesthesia, shunt obstruction and infection
  amongst others make this not without its risks.

Optic nerve sheath fenestration
Fewer complications than lumboperitoneal shunt,
  but the procedure may cause blindness in the
  treated eye. Recent reports suggest that the
  early improvement following this procedure
  may not be sustained.
Patients must be followed up for several years
  with visual field perimetry in case of treatment
  failure.

PROGNOSIS

Permanent visual loss may be present in 50%
and this may cause significant morbidity in as
many as 10%. Although the symptoms of benign
intracranial hypertension tend to recede with
time, the raised pressure may persist.

QUESTION SPOTTING

Grey case
The typical question will include an obese
women aged 20–40 years with visual symptoms
or headaches. Dural sinus thrombosis and
intracranial mass should be actively looked for.

Data interpretation
Unlikely to appear in this section.

MYASTHENIA GRAVIS

Muscle weakness and fatiguability that is caused by autoimmune anti-acetylcholine receptor antibodies which block the postsynaptic receptors at the neuromuscular junction as well as reducing their numbers. Although the mechanism is now well understood, the aetiology is not. There is a strong association with thymic abnormalities. Most are thymic hyperplasia, while the rest are thymomas. Thymectomy results in clinical improvement in many patients. A viral trigger has been suggested but has never been proven. The most promising theory is that the antibodies are induced by an infectious agent that in part resembles the acetylcholine receptor causing cross reactivity.

Onset is bimodal, with a peak in the 2nd and 3rd decades affecting mostly women, and a late smaller peak in the 6th and 7th decades mostly affecting men.

SYMPTOMS

Muscle weakness and fatiguability
Double vision (only presenting feature in 15%)
Nasal speech
Choking
Difficulty chewing
Difficulty swallowing
Difficulty breathing – may be life threatening.
 (myasthenic crisis)

SIGNS

Diplopia
Ptosis
Nasal speech
Flat facial features
Proximal limb weakness – may affect the neck
 extensors
Muscle fatiguability

INVESTIGATIONS

FBC
Normal

U + Es
Normal

LFTs
Normal

ESR normal
CRP normal
ANA may be positive
Rheumatoid factor may be positive
Thyroid function tests – may demonstrate
 autoimmune thyroid disease
Fasting blood glucose – may indicate diabetes

Chest X-ray
Thymic enlargement

CT or MRI chest
Enlargement of thymus

Spirometry
Vital capacity ↓ is an indication for
 plasmapheresis

DIAGNOSIS

Anti-acetylcholine receptor antibodies are highly
 specific, but only 85% sensitive (less in pure
 ocular disease)
Edrophonium (Tensilon) test should show clear
 improvement
Single fibre EMG with repetitive stimulation
 shows fatiguability

ASSOCIATIONS

There is an association with HLA B8 and HLA
DR3 group autoimmune conditions especially:
Graves' disease
SLE
Rheumatoid arthritis
Pernicious anaemia

TREATMENT

Anticholinesterase drugs
Pyridostigmine. Cholinergic side effects include
 diarrhoea and colic which may be reduced by
 simultaneous administration of propantheline.

Thymectomy
Generally accepted that removal of thymus gives
 benefit to most patients with generalized
 myasthenia, and have evidence of thymic
 enlargement. Patients may show initial
 deterioration postoperatively, and so surgery
 should only be carried out electively in

139

specialized centre. Plasmapheresis preoperatively should be carried out if the vital capacity is less than 2 L.

Steroids

Indicated in moderate to severe generalized disease and ocular myasthenia. Patients should be hospitalized due to common initial deterioration, which can be minimized by incrementing the dose.

Azathioprine

Indicated if steroids fail or as a steroid sparing agent. Action is very slow to begin, and may take up to a year to exert an effect.

Cyclosporin

Same efficacy as azathioprine, but faster onset of action. This is balanced against frequent side effects and high cost.

Immunoglobulins and plasma exchange

Short-term treatment for myasthenic crisis or pre-operatively. Exerts a rapid effect, but lasts only a few weeks. Immunoglobulin may have longer effects and does not require central venous access but is very expensive. Mechanism of action is not known.

DIFFERENTIAL DIAGNOSIS

Congenital myasthenic syndromes – rare
Drug induced myasthenia, e.g. penicillamine (induces autoimmune myasthenia) or aminoglycosides, quinines, procainamide (exacerbation of myasthenia that recovers on drug withdrawal)

Hyperthyroidism – thyroid function should always be screened
Lambert-Eaton syndrome – may involve autonomic and sensory systems and rarely the extraorbital muscles
Guillain-Barré syndrome
Botulism
Progressive external ophthalmoplegia
Cranial masses causing ophthalmoplegia or cranial nerve palsies

PROGNOSIS

Variable. If confined to the extraocular muscles, the prognosis is excellent.
Young women tend to relapse early after thymectomy and elderly patients tend not to have remission at all.

QUESTION SPOTTING

Grey case

Mostly suited to this type of question. Usually the differential is with Guillain-Barré syndrome, or botulism. Look for clues such as worsening in the evenings. Initial muscle power is normal, and the reflexes are normal. There are never any sensory symptoms.

Data interpretation

Not suited to this type of question.

MULTIPLE SCLEROSIS

Despite intensive research, much remains unknown about multiple sclerosis, but the main areas of investigation include lipid metabolism, autoimmunity and infection. The disease process centres around the destruction of myelin in the central nervous system (without involvement of the peripheral nervous system). This process may either be a direct immunological attack on the myelin sheath itself or on the oligodendrocyte cells which produce the myelin. These areas of demyelination known as plaques occur mainly in a perivenous and periventricular distribution and vary in size from 1 mm to 4 cm.

The pattern of disease is highly variable, making diagnosis and treatment difficult, but certain disease patterns seem to occur. The most common is the relapsing/remitting type – others include the acute, progressive and benign forms. It is also likely that a subclinical form exists since demyelinated plaques can be seen at autopsy.

SYMPTOMS

Eye pain
Blurred vision
Double vision
Vertigo
Dizziness
Numbness
Weakness
Paraesthesia
Urinary retention or incontinence
Tremor – rare
Facial pain – trigeminal neuralgia – rare
Loss of memory – late

SIGNS

Reduced acuity
Blurred optic disc
Pale optic disc – starts in the temporal region of the discs
Nystagmus
Internuclear ophthalmoplegia
Increased muscular tone
Reduced muscular power
Increased reflexes and upgoing plantars
Positive Lhermitte's sign – tingling in the spine or limbs on neck flexion
Partial Brown-Séquard syndrome

INVESTIGATIONS

FBC
Normal

U + Es
Normal

LFTs
Normal

Vitamin B12 and folate normal

DIAGNOSIS

CSF
Protein ↑
Lymphocytes ↑
IgG ↑ (oligoclonal bands on electrophoresis).
  Occasional ↑ IgM or IgA.

Since low levels of immunoglobulin are seen in the CSF, contamination by blood is easy, and so it is useful to compare CSF with serum.

MRI
Multiple high signal plaques, particularly in the brain stem, and periventricular regions (See Fig. 12). More sensitive than CT and now in routine use to assist in the diagnosis. Can be used to predict which patients with clinically isolated syndromes will progress to multiple sclerosis.

Electrophysiological studies
Visual, auditory and somatic sensory evoked potentials typically show delay without loss of amplitude (Fig. 13).

DIFFERENTIAL DIAGNOSIS

Brain stem and optic lesions may be seen in
Sarcoid
Neurosyphilis
SLE
Behçet's disease

Spinal cord lesions may be confused with
Cervical myelopathy with spondylosis (which may co-exist)
Spinal cord compression
Subacute combined degeneration of the spinal cord

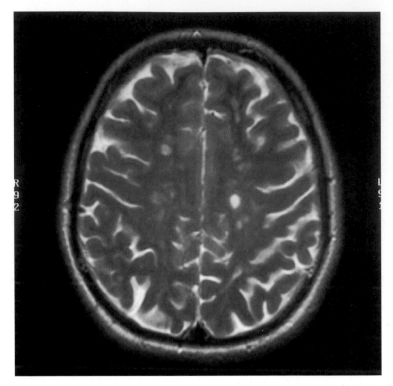

Fig. 12. Multiple sclerosis. T2 weight MRI of brain showing multiple areas of high attenuation typical of multiple sclerosis.

Other diseases which may cause diagnostic confusion
Recurrent thromboembolic disease
Friedreich's ataxia
Acute disseminated encephalomyelitis
Neuromyelitis optica (Devic's syndrome)
Diffuse scleritis
Central pontine myelinolysis

TREATMENT

Supportive
Support groups
Physiotherapy
Baclofen, diazepam, or tizanidine for spasticity.
Local injection of botulinum toxin can also be used.
Corticosteroids have been shown to speed recovery from an acute relapse, but do not improve long-term outcome. High dose oral steroids are probably as effective as intravenous.
Interferon beta may help in patients with relapsing-remitting disease.
Glatiramer, intravenous immunoglobulins and azathioprine may all be of some benefit, but hyperbaric oxygen, linoleic acid supplements, gluten free diet have all been shown to be ineffective.
Other treatments may be indicated such as sildenafil for erectile dysfunction, oxybutinin for bladder instability, isoniazid or clonazepam for ataxia and carbamazepine or amitriptyline for dysaesthesia.

PROGNOSIS

Highly variable. Life expectancy is typically 20–30 years from onset of symptoms.

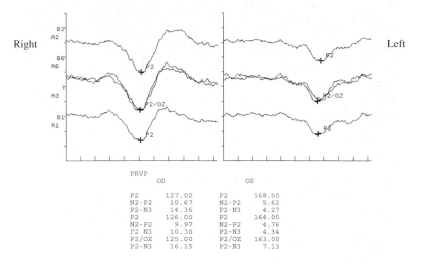

Fig. 13. **Multiple sclerosis.** The visual evoked potentials show delay on the right side with normal waveform and amplitude, and severe delay on the left.

Visual Evoked Potential (Pattern)
   P100 Latency

	Right Eye – 02 = 127.0 ms	Left Eye – 02 = 168.5 ms
	01 = 126.0 ms	01 = 164.0 ms

Right: – Delayed, good waveform and amplitude
Left: – Grossly delayed, good waveform and amplitude

20% of patients may have no second relapse after 15 years. 5% may show a rapidly progressive course with death within 5 years.

QUESTION SPOTTING

Grey case

Multiple sclerosis may be present in this form of question as part of the differential cause of complex neurological features. Remember it is the most common cause of neurological deficit that is separated in both place and time. It should always be considered as a diagnosis in patients presenting with painful blurring of one eye.

Data interpretation

Most likely to be asked to interpret some sensory evoked potentials.

MYOTONIC DYSTROPHY

Autosomal dominant disorder caused by increased trinucleotide repeats (AGC repeat) on chromosome 19q. The number of repeats may increase from generation to generation giving rise to increasingly severe disease (anticipation). The muscles involved are particularly those of the face, neck and distal extremities, but with increasing severity, more central muscles, including proximal limb muscles, muscles of the pharynx and larynx, and even the diaphragm may be involved. Myotonia is the inability of a contracted muscle group to quickly relax. Tends to present between 10 and 30 years of age, although features may be seen in the first decade.

CLINICAL FEATURES

Muscular features
Wasting of the involved muscles – gives a typical expressionless 'hatchet face' due to wasting of the temporalis, masseters and sternomastoids (prone to recurrent dislocation of jaw)
Bilateral ptosis
Myotonia
Weakness in the hands and wrists
Weakness of ankle dorsiflexion results in foot drop
Dysarthria
Dysphagia
Diaphragmatic weakness may lead to respiratory insufficiency
Diplopia if extraocular muscles involved (rare)

Endocrine
Impaired glucose tolerance or frank diabetes mellitus.
Males: impotence, gonadal failure
Females: irregular menstruation and infertility

Cardiac
Conduction defects
AV block
RBBB
LBBB

Mitral valve prolapse
Cardiomyopathy
Sudden death

Gastrointestinal
Constipation
Diarrhoea
Abdominal cramps
Gallstones

Other
Frontal baldness
Cataracts – stellate
Somnolence
Progressive dementia
Hyperostosis of skull vault and small sella turcica
Abnormal immunoglobulin production may lead to increased infections

INVESTIGATIONS

FBC
Normal

U + Es
Normal

LFTs
Normal
Creatinine kinase – normal c.f. myositis
May slightly ↑ late in the disease
IgG often ↓
Thyroid function normal

ECG
Conduction abnormalities including AV block, RBBB, LBBB

EEG
Often abnormal

DIAGNOSIS

EMG
Myotonic discharges – repetitive single motor unit potentials and low amplitude short duration, polyphasic motor unit potentials.

Muscle biopsy
Typically type 1 muscle fibre atrophy.
Occasional type 2 hypertrophy. Necrosis and degeneration are notably absent.

DIFFERENTIAL DIAGNOSIS

Muscular dystrophies – Becker's muscular dystrophy, facioscapulohumeral muscular dystrophy

Polymyositis
Hypothyroidism

TREATMENT

Supportive – splints for foot drop.
   Myotonia may be treated with phenytoin.
   Methylphenidate may be used for
      hypersomnolence.
   Cataract extraction if visual impairment.

QUESTION SPOTTING

Grey case

Although more suited for PACES, myotonic
dystrophy may appear in the written section. The typical patient will be in their teens or twenties
and will usually present with weakness or muscle
stiffness (rather than myotonia). Look out for
cardiac involvement and cataracts.

Data interpretation

You may be asked to interpret an EMG report for
this disorder.

FRIEDREICH'S ATAXIA

Autosomal recessive disease caused by expansion of trinucleotide repeats in chromosome 9q. The size of the repeat section correlates with the age of onset, and the presence of cardiomyopathy and diabetes. The disease is characterized by neurodegeneration and cardiomyopathy. The neurodegeneration is thought to begin in the dorsal root ganglia, with loss of sensory neurones. Later, axonal sensory and motor neuropathy occur, with loss of the spinal tracts. There is cerebellar involvement with atrophy. Cognitive function is preserved throughout the disease. Mean age of onset is 14 years, with presentation usually before 25 years of age.

CLINICAL FEATURES

Neurological
Ataxia affecting gait and stance
Areflexia of legs (very rarely increased reflexes)
Loss of vibration and position sense
Extensor plantars (65%)
Progressive muscular weakness and wasting with normal or decreased tone
Dysarthria (late) with hesitation and scanning speech
Optic atrophy (30%)
Retinitis pigmentosa
Sensorineural deafness
Bladder dysfunction
Flexor spasms (rare)
Loss of pain and light touch (10%)
Oculomotor disturbance – fixation instability, ↓ vestibulo-ocular reflex, jerky pursuit
Nystagmus (30%)

Non-neurological
Hypertrophic cardiomyopathy
Diabetes mellitus (10%)
Skeletal deformities (90%), e.g. pes cavus, equinovarus deformity, scoliosis

INVESTIGATIONS

FBC
Normal

U + Es
Normal
Glucose may be ↑

LFTs
Normal

Nerve conduction
Sensory potentials – reduced/absent (sensory axonal neuropathy)
Motor potentials – ↓ response or slowed conduction time
Visual, auditory and somatosensory evoked potentials show delay or absent potentials

ECG
T wave inversion and non-specific changes

Echocardiography
Interventricular septal hypertrophy
Left ventricular hypertrophy
Reduced left ventricular dimensions

MRI
May confirm cerebellar atrophy

DIAGNOSIS

Clinical features
PCR can show homozygosity for GAA repeat sequence

DIFFERENTIAL DIAGNOSIS

Hereditary motor-sensory neuropathies: (no oculomotor disturbance, no cardiomyopathy, and no dysarthria)
Refsum's disease
Vitamin E deficiency ataxia
Ataxia-telangiectasia
Abetalipoproteinaemia
Multiple sclerosis

TREATMENT

Physiotherapy
Supportive treatments including wheelchairs when required
Oral hypoglycaemics for diabetes
Corrective surgery for skeletal deformities

PROGNOSIS

Wheelchair bound within 10–12 years, and death within 35 years is usual.

QUESTION SPOTTING

Grey case

Although more typical for the PACES, Friedreich's ataxia may present an adult grey case. The typical patient will be young and should show the cardinal features of progressive ataxia, lower limb areflexia, reduced position or vibration sense in the lower limbs and dysarthria within 5 years of the onset of ataxia. These features are definitive for Friedreich's ataxia.

Note that Friedreich's ataxia is one of the causes of extensor plantars with absent tendon reflexes at the ankle.

Data interpretation

Unlikely to appear here, but may present with some evoked potential reports.

GUILLAIN-BARRÉ SYNDROME

An acute polyneuropathy, usually demyelinating, which is thought to be caused by an autoimmune process triggered by a recent infection.

Agents which can trigger Guillain-Barré include:

Campylobacter jejuni
HIV
CMV
EBV
Enteroviruses
Mycoplasma species
Other upper respiratory tract pathogens.

In 60% of cases, a prodromal illness (URTI or diarrhoea) precedes onset of symptoms by 1–2 weeks.

SYMPTOMS

Limb weakness (usually starts in legs, and ascends)
Pain (usually in back)
Numbness, paraesthesia (usually distal)
Dizziness due to autonomic neuropathy
Constipation due to autonomic neuropathy
Nausea due to autonomic neuropathy
Sweating due to autonomic neuropathy

SIGNS

Tachycardia or bradycardia
Hypertension or hypotension (especially on standing)
Reduced muscle tone
Limb weakness
Reduced light touch / vibration / joint position sense
Reduced reflexes (may be preserved at first)
Papilloedema
Cranial nerve involvement (usually VII, less commonly bulbar, rarely ocular)

NB. Miller-Fisher variant (3%): Ataxia, ophthalmoplegia plus reduced reflexes. Power is relatively spared in limbs

Diffuse cranial nerve involvement may also occur (polyneuritis cranialis)

INVESTIGATIONS

FBC
Usually normal

U + Es
Usually normal

LFTs
ALT $\uparrow$ (33%)
GGT $\uparrow$ (33%)

CK may be raised
ESR raised

Autoantibodies
GM1 positive in 25%. Associated with worse outcome
GQ1B associated with Miller-Fisher variant and ophthalmoplegia

CSF
Protein raised (may be normal in first 2 weeks)
WCC often normal. Almost always <50 lymphocytes/cm

Nerve conduction studies usually show a demyelinating pattern. Some patients may display axonal loss with little or no evidence of demyelination.
PFTs may show reduced FVC.

DIAGNOSIS

Is primarily on clinical grounds. The presence of demyelination on nerve conduction studies, and a high protein with low cell count in the CSF, are corroborating factors.

DIFFERENTIAL DIAGNOSIS

Drugs
E.g. neuromuscular junction blockers

Autoimmune
Myasthenia gravis
Eaton-Lambert syndrome
Vasculitis
Multiple sclerosis

Metabolic
Porphyria
Lead poisoning
Low K^+
High Mg^{++}

Toxic
Snake / scorpion / fish toxins
Tick paralysis

Infection
Polio
Botulism

Other
Myopathy of critically ill (found in intensive care patients)

COMPLICATIONS

Respiratory paralysis
Arrhythmias / cardiovascular instability
Pressure sores
Thromboembolic disease

TREATMENT

IV immunoglobulin for 5 days, unless illness mild or improving at diagnosis. Plasma exchange is an alternative
Subcutaneous heparin
Monitor FVC closely. If FVC <20 ml/Kg (approx 1.5 L), consider elective intubation (needed in 25% of all patients)
Physiotherapy and later, occupational therapy
Analgesia for pain

PROGNOSIS

70–80% recover fully, although this may take months. Recovery usually starts within 2 to 4 weeks of onset.
5–10% die, usually of cardiovascular problems, infection or thromboembolism.
15% have some degree of significant residual disability.

QUESTION SPOTTING

Grey case
Usually occurs as a patient with rapid onset of weakness. Clues to the diagnosis are:

Relative sparing of the eye muscles
High CSF protein
Prominent autonomic symptoms
Prodromal illness

Data interpretation
Usually as results from a sample of CSF. Protein is usually high, with near normal WCC and normal glucose. Protein may be up to 3–4 g/L; if it is above 4 g/L, consider Froin's syndrome (spinal block).

NORMAL PRESSURE HYDROCEPHALUS

Normal pressure hydrocephalus (NPH) is hydrocephalus in the absence of raised intracranial pressure (defined as 15 mmHg intracranial pressure). NPH may be caused by intracranial haemorrhage, head injury, intracranial surgery and meningitis, but 60% have no known cause. The mechanism of the disease is thought to be reduced reabsorption of CSF by the arachnoid villi. Despite the name, the intracranial pressure is not completely normal. There are transient increases in pressure, which may cause the ventricular enlargement.

The disease is rare in the under-sixties. However it may occur as a consequence of one of the causes mentioned above. NPH is thought to account for as many as 5% of dementia in the older population, but its true prevalence is unknown.

CLINICAL FEATURES

Triad of (tend to occur in the given order):
Gait disturbance – slow, ataxic and wide based with short steps.
Dementia – affects all function including attention, memory, execution
Urinary incontinence

Other features include:
Apathy
Tremor (postural)
Increased tone in the legs
Hyper-reflexia of the legs.
Impairment of fine movement like handwriting
Dysphasia and apraxias are rare, cf. Alzheimer's disease.

INVESTIGATIONS

FBC
Normal

U + Es
Normal

LFTs
Normal

CSF
Normal composition

EEG
Normal
PET scanning using glucose markers shows hypometabolism (different pattern from Alzheimer's disease).

DIAGNOSIS

Intracranial pressure (ICP) monitoring shows peaks of pressure (B waves) over a background of normal pressure. Drainage of 20–30 ml of CSF may cause clinical improvement.
CT/MRI head shows hydrocephalus with no cause for obstruction to CSF flow. On T2 signal MRI periventricular oedema may be seen.

DIFFERENTIAL DIAGNOSIS

Alzheimer's disease – not associated with gait dysfunction.
Multi-infarct dementia – neuroimaging should show evidence of infarction or ischaemia.
Obstructive hydrocephalus.

TREATMENT

Acetazolamide or digoxin may be used (limited success).
Lumbar puncture drainage of CSF.
Ventricular shunting if recent onset dementia, no evidence of multi-infarct dementia, large numbers of B waves on ICP monitoring and no evidence of passive ventricular enlargement secondary to cerebral atrophy. Shunt complication rates are up to 30% and include subdural haematoma, epilepsy, shunt infection and occlusion.

PROGNOSIS

Better prognosis if cause is known and recent onset and if shunting procedure performed. Long history, cerebral atrophy and vascular disease are all bad predictors of outcome.

QUESTION SPOTTING

Grey case

Unlikely to get the classic triad handed to you on a plate! Remember the order of occurrence.

Exclude other causes of confusion in the elderly.

Data interpretation

Unlikely to appear in this section.

VARIANT CREUTZFELDT-JAKOB DISEASE (vCJD)

Variant Creutzfeldt-Jakob disease is a disease caused by prion protein (PrP) and is characterized by spongiform encephalopathy. Although this onset of a new clinical syndrome has been closely linked with the outbreak of bovine spongiform encephalopathy (BSE), which peaked in incidence in the UK in 1992, no absolute proof of a causal relationship has yet been found. PrP occurs in normal people as an alpha-helical structure but in vCJD, PrP undergoes post-translational change to a beta-sheet form. This is resistant to proteases and accumulates in neural cells, disrupting function and leading to vacuolization and cell death.

Variant CJD is still rare. Between 1995 and December 1999 there have been 49 deaths attributed to variant CJD in the UK. All patients had eaten meat (although one became a strict vegetarian in 1992). The incubation period is believed to be at least 4 years. The disease appears to have a long clinical course, with neurological signs appearing several months after first onset of psychiatric disturbance, and death occurring a mean of 7.5 months after onset of neurological signs.

CLINICAL FEATURES

Early
Insomnia.
Weight loss.
Psychiatric disturbance – depressed, apathetic, withdrawn, forgetfulness, depression.
Sensory symptoms – dysaesthesia, paraesthesia.

Late
Neurological disturbance
Ataxia
Dementia
Urinary incontinence
Involuntary movements
Myoclonus
Dysphasia
Dysarthria
Upgaze paresis also seen.

Very late
Immobility
Mutism
Cortical blindness

INVESTIGATIONS

FBC
Normal

U + Es
Normal

LFTs
Normal

EEG
Normal or slow wave activity. Note that none showed the highly typical features (periodic complexes) seen in sporadic CJD

CSF
Protein normal or slightly ↑
Oligoclonal bands negative
Protein 14-3-3 may be positive

CT head
Normal

MRI head
May be normal even late in the disease

Abnormal findings may include:
Mild generalized atrophy
Mildly enlarged ventricles
Areas of high signal in the posterior thalamus on T2 weighted imaging.

DIAGNOSIS

Brain biopsy before or after death.
Tonsil biopsy may provide diagnosis, but low PrP yield

DIFFERENTIAL DIAGNOSIS

Wilson's disease
Schizophrenia
Syphilis
Alcoholism
Multi-infarct dementia and other causes of dementia

Creutzfeldt-Jakob disease (sporadic, familial, iatrogenic)
Gerstmann-Straussler syndrome – extremely rare familial form of spongiform encephalopathy.
Sporadic Creutzfeldt-Jakob disease – age of onset usually 50–65 years old:

Rapid progression of disease such that death may occur within 3 weeks. Few survive longer than 1 year. Psychiatric symptoms are rare. Typical neurological symptoms include early insomnia, nocturnal myoclonus and poor concentration followed by aphasia, cerebellar ataxia, cortical blindness, dementia and fits. Myoclonus becomes prominent. EEG shows typical periodic spikes and slow waves.

TREATMENT

Supportive

QUESTION SPOTTING

Grey case

A new disease form that is topical makes this likely to enter the written examination. The typical patient is young (teens to twenties) with psychiatric disturbance. Sensory symptoms add weight to the diagnosis. Investigations are all normal and the EEG is not diagnostic.

Data interpretation

Unlikely to appear here.

INFECTIOUS DISEASE

SYPHILIS

Syphilis is caused by the spirochaete *Treponema pallidum*. Transmission is mostly by sexual contact, and although congenital transmission may occur, it is now very rare. The organism enters the body via an abrasion during sexual contact, and there is an incubation period of about 3 weeks. The infection follows a typical pattern, but progression may halt at any stage. Tissue damage is caused by obliterative endarteritis. The disease incidence fell throughout the 20th century until around 1985 when an increase was noted, thought to be associated with the spread of HIV. Late stages of syphilis are still very rare, probably due to the use of antibiotics in non-related conditions.

Women show milder early symptoms (especially during pregnancy) and are less likely to develop neurosyphilis or cardiovascular syphilis.

CLINICAL FEATURES

Primary syphilis

Development of small painless papule, which ulcerates to form a painless, oval ulcer (the chancre). The site is usually the penis in heterosexual men, the anal canal in homosexual men, and the vulva or labia in women. More rarely, the cervix may be involved or other sites such as the lip, mouth, or hand. The ulcer is highly infectious.

Secondary syphilis

Secondary syphilis occurs 4–6 weeks after the chancre, lasts 2–6 weeks and resolves without any residual signs.

Symptoms

Headaches and neck stiffness – due to low grade meningitis
Slight fever
Malaise
Arthralgia
Myalgia
Rash – symmetrical, non-itchy, commonly on the trunk. It also may involve the palms, soles or face, where it should raise immediate suspicion of syphilis
Alopecia – rare
Laryngitis – rare
Bone pain due to periostitis – rare

Jaundice and abdominal pain secondary to hepatitis – rare

Signs

Generalized painless lymphadenopathy
Condylomata lata – papules occurring in moist areas, such as the perineum
Buccal snail track ulcers
Uveitis – seen in both secondary and tertiary syphilis
Nephrotic syndrome – very rare

Tertiary syphilis

Occurs after 2–20 year latent period. Patients are generally non-infectious, but may remain infectious (e.g. women may give birth to a child with congenital syphilis).

Cutaneous gumma

Inflammatory nodules which break down to become ulcers. These heal with scarring and are typically hypopigmented in the centre and hyperpigmented around the edges.

Mucosal gumma

Destructive ulcers that involve the palate, pharynx and nasal septum causing perforation. Involvement of the tongue may lead to leukoplakia, and eventually malignancy.

Osteoperiostitis

Thickening and irregularity of the long bones with severe pain

Liver

Irregular hepatomegaly secondary to multiple gummas

Eyes

Uveitis
Choroidoretinitis
Optic atrophy

Stomach

Gummatous infiltration

Lungs

Gummas may occur

Testis

Smooth painless enlargement secondary to gummas

Blood

Paroxysmal nocturnal haemoglobinuria

Cardiovascular syphilis

Aortitis (asymptomatic) – causes calcification of ascending aorta

Aortic aneurysm formation (saccular and often painful)

Aortic regurgitation

Coronary artery ostial stenosis

Neurosyphilis

Meningovascular syphilis – acute meningitis occurs early with cranial nerve palsies (may be bilateral) and papilloedema. Meningeal irritation may be minimal. Later, hydrocephalus, fits, strokes, radiculopathy and amyotrophic meningomyelitis occur.

'General paresis of the insane'(GPI) – progressive dementia, with personality change which eventually leads to motor involvement and paralysis. Delusions occur but the classic grandiose delusions are actually rare.

Tabes dorsalis – lightning pains, leg ataxia, and bladder dysfunction is the classic triad. However, Argyll-Robertson pupils, loss of vibration and position sense, and upper limb pathology may all occur. Charcot joints occur.

INVESTIGATIONS

FBC

Hb may be ↓ if paroxysmal nocturnal haemoglobinuria

U + Es

Normal

LFTs

AST may be ↑

ALT may be ↑

Bilirubin may be ↑

ALP may be ↑

CSF

Protein ↑ (>0.4 g/L)

WCC ↑ (5–50/mm³ CSF)

VDRL positive (in only 50%)

TPHA and FTA-ABS positive (but remain positive long after successful treatment)

DIAGNOSIS

Serology

Non-specific

RPR – rapid plasma reagin test

VDRL – Venereal Disease Research Laboratory test

Both of these tests have a high false positive rate (e.g. SLE or pregnancy) but false positive titres are usually lower than titres seen in syphilis infection. Both tests usually become negative following successful treatment as their titre follows disease activity.

Specific

TPHA – *Treponema pallidum* haemagglutination test

FTA-ABS – indirect fluorescent test

Both of these tests are highly specific for the *Treponema* group but cannot differentiate one species from another (e.g. Yaws). They do not mirror disease activity. TPHA is the most specific test in modern use, but is not as sensitive as FTA-ABS. Both tests remain positive long after successful treatment.

DIFFERENTIAL DIAGNOSIS

Primary syphilis

Chancroid

Genital herpes

Drug reactions

Erosive balanitis

Tertiary syphilis

Gumma

Sarcoid

Tuberculosis

Leprosy

Lymphogranuloma venereum

Reticulosis

Donovanosis

Osteoperiostitis

Paget's disease

Osteomyelitis

Carcinoma

Leprosy

Causes of a false positive VDRL

Autoimmune disease – especially SLE

Pregnancy
Drug addicts
Leprosy
Old age
Antiphospholipid syndrome

TREATMENT

Procaine penicillin for 10–14 days
(tetracycline/erythromycin if true penicillin
allergy). The Jarisch-Herxheimer reaction may
occur 4–12 h following first injection in 50% of
primary syphilis, 90% of secondary and 25% of
tertiary. However, this reaction may cause
irreversible progression of clinical features in
tertiary disease. The reaction does not relate to
dose of penicillin. Steroids may be given to
reduce the reaction.

Trace sexual contacts (how far back depends on
stage of disease)

QUESTION SPOTTING

Grey case

Although syphilis is still rare in the UK, the
incidence is rising and there is a strong rise in the
HIV positive population. Syphilis may come up
in this section in conjunction with another
disease such as HIV or as a cause of unusual
cardiac/neurological symptoms and signs.
Another cause of extensor plantars with absent
ankle reflexes.

Data interpretation

Watch out for the serology and think of other
causes of a positive VDRL.

BRUCELLOSIS

Infection by *Brucella* spp, a genus of intracellular gram negative bacilli. Four species are known to cause human disease:

B. melitensis: sheep, goats
B. abortus: cattle
B. suis: pigs
B. canis: dogs

The infection has an incubation period of 1 to 3 weeks. Sources of infection include unpasteurized milk, soft cheese (e.g. goat's), animal faeces and urine. Routes of infection are inhalation, ingestion or via broken skin. At risk groups include animal workers, e.g. farmers and vets.

SYMPTOMS

Fever (not always 'undulant') (90%)
Sweats (90%)
Myalgia (90%)
Joint and back pain (85%)
Headache (80%)
Weight loss (70%)
Anorexia
Constipation (45%)
Abdominal pain (45%)
Cough (25%)
Testicular pain (20% men)
Rash (15%)
Diarrhoea

SIGNS

Spine tenderness (50%)
Arthritis (40%)
Lymphadenopathy (30%)
Splenomegaly (25%)
Pallor
Hepatomegaly (20%)
Epididymo-orchitis (20%)

CNS signs (rare)
Meningoencephalitis
Cranial nerve palsies
Radiculopathy
Hemiplegia

Cardiac murmur – rare
Jaundice – rare
Signs of pneumonia – rare

Other manifestations
Cardiac
Endocarditis
Myocarditis
Pericarditis
Aortic root abscess

Gastrointestinal
Colitis
Peritonitis
Pancreatitis
Hepatitis (usually mild)

Skin
Subcutaneous nodules
Erythema nodosum
Maculopapular rash
Purpura
Ulceration

Eye
Endophthalmitis
Conjunctivitis
Keratitis

Neurological
Guillain-Barré syndrome
Transverse myelitis
Cerebral abscess

Joints
Reactive arthritis, usually large joint,
    polyarticular
Septic arthritis
Spondylitis
Osteomyelitis

INVESTIGATIONS

FBC
Hb may be ↓ (chronic infection)
WCC usually normal or neutropenic
Platelets usually normal

U + Es
Normal

LFTs
Albumin may be ↓
AST mildly ↑
ALP mildly ↑
Bilirubin mildly ↑

INR, APTT usually normal. DIC is rare
ESR ↑

CXR occasionally shows consolidation, hilar
  lymphadenopathy or effusions.
Joint fluid shows elevated neutrophil count. High
  protein, low glucose. Organism cultured in
  50%.
Urine positive for culture in 50%.
CSF in meningoencephalitis, shows elevated
  lymphocyte count, high protein, normal or low
  glucose, raised oligoclonal Ig. Organism can
  be cultured from CSF.
Organ biopsy may show granulomas, which may
  caseate.

DIAGNOSIS

Blood cultures positive in 50% (must incubate
  for 6 weeks)
Bone marrow cultures positive in 50–70%

Serology (agglutination tests)
Fourfold rise in titre over 4 weeks
or >1 : 160 (non-endemic area)
or >1 : 640 (endemic area)

Raised IgM titres denote recent infection. Raised
IgG titres denote active infection. Assays can
cross react with cholera and tularemia.

DIFFERENTIAL DIAGNOSIS

Any cause of a PUO, especially granulomatous
  diseases, e.g. TB, sarcoid
Metastatic malignancy
Vasculitides
SBE

Pyogenic abscess
Typhoid

TREATMENT

Tetracycline (e.g. doxycycline) plus
  aminoglycoside (e.g. IM streptomycin).
  Therapy is continued for 1 month, then
  tetracyclines plus either rifampicin or co-
  trimoxazole is continued for 2 months.
  Relapse rate is 7%.
Neurobrucellosis: add in rifampicin at start.

NB: Jarisch-Herxheimer reaction may occur on
starting antibiotics.

PROGNOSIS

Good recovery when treated; untreated, illness
may persist in a chronic form for many years.
Neurological deficit may occur, and destruction
of heart valves occurs with endocarditis.

QUESTION SPOTTING

Grey case
Clues to the diagnosis are:

Pyrexia of unknown origin
Patient has been abroad (especially Malta) and
  drunk unpasteurized milk
Back pain as a prominent symptom
Fever with a low neutrophil count
Granulomas on organ biopsy

Data interpretation
Unlikely to occur in this section.

TYPHOID FEVER

Typhoid fever is caused by the organism *Salmonella typhi*, a Gram negative bacillus. The source is usually faecal contamination, but may be from sputum, vomitus or other body fluid. Incubation is from 8 days to 3 weeks. After this, the organism invades the blood stream via the thoracic duct and causes systemic disease. Organs particularly affected are the liver, spleen, gut, bone marrow and gall bladder. Untreated the disease lasts about 4 weeks. Initially fever may be the only symptom, but as the disease progresses, so complications are more likely.

CLINICAL FEATURES

Early
Symptoms
Fever (up to 39–40°), gradual onset, and rarely causes rigors and very little diurnal variation – 'ramping' continuous fever
Headache
Weight loss
Malaise
Anorexia
Myalgia
Arthralgia
Epistaxis is common early on
Constipation is classical symptom unlike infection with other *Salmonella*, but most patients also have loose stool at some point
Nausea and vomiting

Signs
Bradycardia relative to the fever is typical

Later – 1 week
Symptoms
Cough
Bloody diarrhoea with ileal ulceration or fulminant colitis.

Signs
Rash – rose spots on trunk
Abdominal distension
Mild splenomegaly may occur.

Severe late – 2 weeks +
Delirium
Tremor
Ataxia
Coma
Death

INVESTIGATIONS

FBC
Hb normal or ↓ (normal MCV)
WCC often normal or ↓
Platelets often ↓

U + Es
Na ↓
K ↓
Urea and creatinine ↑ if nephritis

LFTs
AST normal or ↑
ALT normal or ↑
Bilirubin normal or ↑
ALP normal or ↑
Albumin normal or ↓
ESR ↑
Clotting frequently prolonged
Serology (Widal reaction) usually rising antibody titre to O and H antigens.

DIAGNOSIS

Positive culture for *Salmonella typhi* from bone marrow (highly sensitive – days 7–10 best), blood (80% sensitive – days 7–10 best), rose spots (70% sensitive), and urine/stool (low sensitivity – positive in 2nd–3rd weeks).

COMPLICATIONS

Gastrointestinal
Intestinal perforation and haemorrhage (<5% and usually terminal ileum)
Hepatitis, cholecystitis, pancreatitis

Cardiovascular
Pancarditis
Asymptomatic ECG changes
Sudden cardiac death
DVT

Respiratory
Pneumonia
Bronchitis
Respiratory tract ulceration

Neurological
Delirium
Psychosis
Depression

Meningo-encephalitis
Focal neurological signs
Guillain-Barré syndrome

Renal
Nephritis

Haematological
Deranged clotting
Anaemia
Haemolysis
HUS

TREATMENT

Fluid management
Antipyretics
Observation for complications
Antibiotics – ciprofloxacin 1st line or
    amoxycillin/choramphenicol/co-trimoxazole
    2nd line though resistance increasing
Dexamethasone has a place in severe typhoid
    (shock or coma) where mortality reaches as
    high as 50%
Surgery if intestinal perforation

Carrier status
Excretion of *S. typhi* in asymptomatic individuals
for 3 months after treatment is relatively
common. Up to 3% of patients continue to
excrete *S. typhi* in their stool for more than
1 year and are defined as chronic carriers (and
may excrete bacilli indefinitely). The gallbladder
is usually the site of persistent infection. Urinary
carriage is associated with *schistosoma* infection
and nephrolithiasis. Acute typhoid may recur,
and there is an increased incidence of
cholangiocarcinoma. Treatment of carriers is
with 4 weeks of ciprofloxacin and
cholecystectomy is rarely required.

Prophylaxis
Prevention with one of the three available
    vaccines is recommended for travellers to
    endemic areas.
Treatment of water by heat or chemicals and
    careful hygiene are essential.

QUESTION SPOTTING

Grey case
Typhoid fever is one of the diseases that must be
excluded in travellers returning home from
tropical or less well developed countries (along
with malaria). The cardinal symptoms are fever
and headache. Rash, bradycardia, constipation
are clues. Blood results may resemble legionella
but a ↑ WCC occurs in typhoid only in
complications such as perforation.

Data interpretation
Less likely to appear in this section, but the
blood results with a short clinical history may
lead to the diagnosis of typhoid.

TUBERCULOSIS

Caused by the organism *Mycobacterium tuberculosis*, tuberculosis (TB) is still a major cause of morbidity and mortality worldwide. Rarely, the disease may be caused by other mycobacteria, such as *Mycobacterium bovis* or *Mycobacterium avium-intracellulare* (MAI). Although primarily an infection of the lungs, the disease can spread to involve virtually any other organ. Spread is usually by droplet and is particularly prevalent in overcrowding, poor social conditions and poor nutrition. More recently, an increase in TB has been seen in the HIV positive population.

The classic pathology of TB is the caseating granuloma. The necrotic centre is surrounded by epithelioid cells and Langhans' giant cells with multiple nuclei. The granuloma may heal completely, and may calcify. Even calcified lesions may reactivate later if immunity becomes impaired.

The pattern of TB infection may be described as follows:

Primary infection
Usually in childhood.

Usually pulmonary, but occasionally, the primary infection may be at the ileocaecal region of the gastrointestinal tract or the tonsils.

Usually some lymph node spread.

In most people this primary infection heals, but may leave some active bacilli.

Post-primary TB
Primary TB may reactivate during a period of lowered immune resistance, to cause post-primary TB, which may in itself cause progressive or miliary TB.

Progressive TB
Failure of primary or post-primary TB to heal initially leads to progressive TB. This may also occur following reinfection.

Miliary TB
Rarely, primary or post-primary TB may spread via the blood to become widespread. This is miliary TB which is universally fatal untreated. Miliary TB tends to affect younger people, especially young adults.

CLINICAL FEATURES
Primary tuberculosis

Symptoms – rare
Fever
Lethargy
Wheeze
Cough
Conjunctivitis

Signs – rare
Erythema nodosum
Small pleural effusion
Lymphadenopathy

Post-primary

Pulmonary symptoms
Tiredness
Malaise
Fever
Weight loss
Night sweats
Cough
Haemoptysis
Chest pain

Pulmonary signs – rare
Finger clubbing if advanced
Erythema nodosum
Pulmonary crackles may be heard.

Non-pulmonary features

CNS
Meningitis
Tuberculoma

Eye
Phlyctenular conjunctivitis – tuberculous allergic
   hypersensitivity
Iritis
Choroidoretinitis

Cardiac
Pericardial effusion
Cardiac tamponade
Constrictive pericarditis ± pericardial
   calcification

Lymph nodes
Lymph node swelling
Sinus formation

Musculoskeletal
Osteomyelitis
Vertebral collapse (Pott's vertebra)
Psoas abscess

Gastrointestinal
Ascites
Obstruction
Peritonitis

Genitourinary
Renal TB
Cystitis
Dysuria, frequency, sterile pyuria

Epididymitis
Endometrial TB
Salpingitis and tubal abscess

Adrenals
Addison's disease

Skin
Lupus vulgaris
Erythema nodosum

Bone marrow
Anaemia
Thrombocytopenia

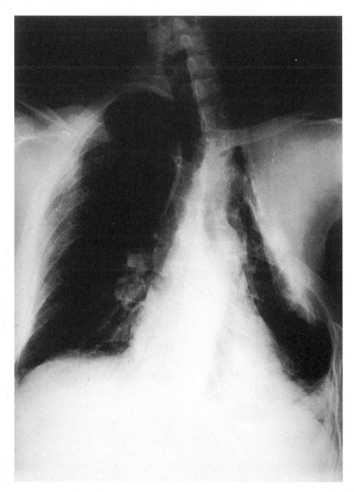

Fig. 14.   TB with previous thoracoplasty. This chest X-ray shows the typical appearances of previous thoracoplasty following TB infection. Although it is rarely done now, there are still many patients alive who have had this procedure.

164

Miliary tuberculosis

Symptoms
High fever
Drenching night sweats
Weight loss
Cough (rare)
Shortness of breath (rare)

Signs
Tachycardia
Anaemia
Hepatomegaly
Splenomegaly
Pulmonary crackles rare until late

INVESTIGATIONS

FBC
Hb ↓
WCC normal or ↑ if miliary TB
Platelets ↓

U + Es
Abnormal if renal TB

LFTs
May show impairment if high tubercle load

ESR ↑
CRP ↑

Chest X-ray
No absolute diagnostic features, but suggestive
 features include:
Nodular shadows in upper lobes
Bilateral upper lobe shadows
Cavitating lesions in upper lobes
Calcified lung lesions
Fibrotic changes
Pleural effusions
Mediastinal enlargement
Previous thoracoplasty – see example chest
 X-ray (Fig. 14)

Immunological
The tuberculin test looks for cell-mediated
response to different concentrations of tuberculin
injected intradermally. More than 10 mm
response at 48–72 h is positive. A positive result
occurs if immunity is present, i.e. previous
infection, current infection, previous BCG. A
large response or response to 1 tuberculin unit is
suggestive of current infection. False negative
tests occur in immune suppression, e.g. miliary
TB, AIDS, lymphoma, sarcoid.
 Sputum examination for acid-fast bacilli with
Ziehl-Nielsen stain or immunofluorescence.
Broncho-alveolar lavage fluid may be used.

DIAGNOSIS

Culture of *Mycobacterium tuberculosis* to
confirm diagnosis and obtain sensitivities.
Culture possible from sputum, broncho-alveolar
lavage, or biopsy of lymph node or pleura.
Early morning urine culture in difficult cases.

COMPLICATIONS

Pneumothorax
Empyema
Tuberculous enteritis
Respiratory failure
Right ventricular failure
Fungal colonization of lung cavities.
Chronic osteomyelitis – see example of spinal
 TB (Pott's disease) (Fig. 15)

TREATMENT

Prevention
BCG vaccination given to 12–13 year olds in UK
if they show a negative tuberculin test. Gives
immunity for approximately 7 years thus
preventing TB when most susceptible to miliary
TB. BCG may also be given to infants of high
risk groups such as Asian immigrants.

Treatment
Standard treatment comprises 2 months of:
pyrazinamide, isoniazid, rifampicin (add
ethambutol if risk of drug resistance). Then
4 months of: isoniazid and rifampicin.
 Full compliance is essential. Taken properly,
this regimen is almost 100% effective. If
compliance is not certain, patients should be
treated as inpatients for the initial 2 months with
the standard triple or quadruple therapy, then
twice weekly streptomycin 1 g i.m. with
15 mg/kg isoniazid and pyridoxine 10 mg
orally, supervised, for a further 10 months.

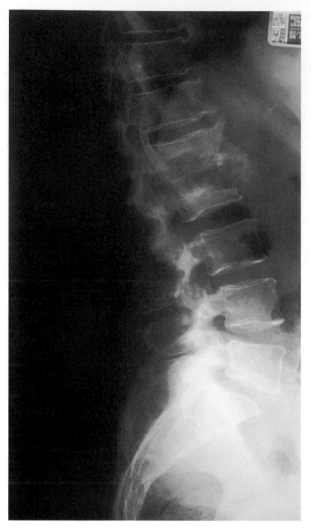

Fig. 15.   Pott's infection of the spine. This lateral spine X-ray shows chronic infection in the L2 disc space. This has expanded and eroded into the adjacent lumbar vertebrae with destruction of the end plates. There is also evidence of a poorly defined soft tissue mass around the joint space.

Common side effects of treatment:

- Rifampicin: orange urine, orange staining to contact lens, oral contraceptive pill inactivation. Hepatitis – stop if bilirubin rises.
- Isoniazid: neuropathy, hepatitis, pyridoxine deficiency, agranulocytosis.
- Pyrazinamide: arthralgia, hepatitis.
- Ethambutol: optic neuritis (colour vision first to be affected and is an indication to stop this treatment).

PROGNOSIS

Cure can be expected for almost any stage of TB infection if therapy is followed correctly, and the organism is not multidrug resistant. Drug resistance is an increasing problem, and requires specialist care. Single drug resistance is common (10%) but multidrug resistance is still rare (0.2%, but this may be an underestimate). Alternative drugs to the standard therapy include:

p-aminosalicylic acid, capreomycin, cycloserine, clarithromycin, ciprofloxacin.

QUESTION SPOTTING

Grey case

Good question for the grey cases. TB should be considered and actively looked for in patients with persistent cough, haemoptysis, pleural pain in the absence of acute illness or pneumothorax, especially if there is any evidence of immunosuppression. The typical patient will be in a high risk group – poor nutrition, alcoholic, ethnic immigrant or immunosuppressed, e.g. AIDS, lymphoma. If the patient has no risk factors, then there must be a history of close contact with active infection.

Data interpretation

Less well suited for this question.

HIV INFECTION

Infection with the human immunodeficiency virus, types 1 and 2. HIV attaches to cells bearing the CD4 surface protein (mostly T helper lymphocytes and antigen presenting cells), and uses reverse transcriptase to copy the viral RNA into DNA, which then integrates with the host cell genome. Replication and new virus formation then takes place. Over a period of years, the virus slowly erodes the cell mediated immune response, eventually allowing secondary infections and malignancies to occur. The modes of transmission and epidemiology are well covered elsewhere.

FEATURES OF INFECTION

Seroconversion illness (after a 2–6 week incubation)
Fever
Sore throat
Arthralgia
Morbilliform rash
Lymphadenopathy
Candidiasis

Rare manifestations
Guillain-Barré syndrome
Encephalopathy
Seventh cranial nerve palsy
Flare of psoriatic arthropathy

Investigations
FBC may show ↓ lymphocyte count
CD4+ T cell count may be ↓
Atypical lymphocytes on blood film
Antibodies to HIV usually take 3 months to form
HIV PCR and p24 antigen are positive during seroconversion illness

CD4 count 350 to 800 × 10⁶/L
Reactivation of VZV, leading to shingles
Persistent lymphadenopathy

CD4 count 200 to 350 × 10⁶/L
Tuberculosis
TB meningitis
Oral hairy leukoplakia
Candidiasis
Pneumonia (usually conventional organisms)
Non-specific symptoms: fever, myalgia, weight loss, fatigue, diarrhoea

CD4 count <200 × 10⁶/L
Pneumocystis carinii pneumonia
Cerebral toxoplasmosis
Kaposi's sarcoma
Oesophageal candida
Diarrhoea, including *Cryptosporidium*

CD4 count <50 × 10⁶/L
Mycobacterium avium-intracellulare complex (MAC)
Cryptococcal meningitis
Histoplasmosis
CMV retinitis, colitis, oesophagitis, radiculopathy, encephalitis
Non-Hodgkin's lymphoma (high grade, B cell)
Dementia
Progressive multifocal leukoencephalopathy (JC virus)

SYMPTOM COMPLEXES AND PROBABLE CAUSES IN HIV:

Neurological
Depression (30%)
Dementia (30%) – from HIV, PML
Even in asymptomatic disease, CSF often shows raised WBC, protein and IgG

Meningitis
TB
Cryptococcus. Note need to perform India ink staining on CSF
Syphilis
Lymphoma
Other aseptic meningitis

Encephalitis
CMV
HSV
VZV

Space occupying lesions
Toxoplasmosis
Lymphoma

Transverse myelitis (HIV)
Often painless, slowly progressive
Spastic/ataxic paraparesis
Reduced joint position sense, vibration and light touch
Sensory level usually absent

Mononeuritis multiplex (HIV)

Peripheral neuropathy (HIV or medications)

CMV polyradiculopathy
Bowel and bladder dysfunction
Reduced power and reflexes in lower limbs
CSF shows ↑ WCC, ↑ protein and low/normal
  glucose, plus CMV particles

Respiratory
Pneumocystis carinii (see p30)

Pneumonitis
CMV or non-specific
Diagnosis often via BAL at bronchoscopy

Kaposi's sarcoma
Pleural effusion
Cough, SOB, haemoptysis
Respiratory failure may occur
Diagnosis via bronchoscopy or thoracoscopy

Tuberculosis
Cough, sputum, fever
CXR is often atypical in HIV infection
ZN stain is often negative
Tuberculin test is often negative
MAI complex infection often gives systemic
  symptoms

Gastroenterological

Mouth
Aphthous ulcers
Oral hairy leukoplakia

Oesophagus
CMV
HSV
Candida

Diarrhoea
Salmonella; leads to septicaemia in 20–40%
Campylobacter

MAI complex; requires stool culture and jejunal
  biopsy for diagnosis. May lead to a systemic
  illness including fever, weight loss,
  lymphadenopathy and hepatomegaly

Cryptosporidium parvum; may need bowel
  biopsy to diagnose
Microsporidium; found on stool culture
CMV; causes bloody diarrhoea, abdominal pain
  and tenderness, and may lead to perforation or
toxic dilatation. Can be diagnosed on rectal
  biopsy
Sclerosing cholangitis
Pancreatitis (especially as a drug side effect)
Appendicitis (especially from CMV infection)

Dermatology
Multiple warts (HPV)
VZV infection, often of multiple dermatomes.
  May disseminate
Molluscum contagiosum. Often very large
  lesions that do not regress spontaneously
Fungal nail and skin infections
Seborrhoeic dermatitis is increased
Psoriasis. Tends to be more aggressive, and
  psoriatic arthropathy is much more common
Pruritic papular eruption
Eosinophilic folliculitis
Squamous cell carcinoma of the skin is more
  common

Kaposi's sarcoma
Starts as pink macules, then darkens to
  red/purple and becomes raised
Also occur in GI and respiratory tracts
May cause local oedema from lymphatic
  invasion
Common places include genitalia, inner thigh,
  trunk, feet, face, hard palate and conjunctivae
Diagnosed by biopsy. RT, chemo- and
  cryotherapy are all used to treat

Differential diagnosis includes TB, MAI
  complex, *Bartonella* infection

Other problems
Anogenital carcinoma
High grade B cell non-Hodgkin's lymphoma
CMV retinitis; causes reduced visual acuity and
  field loss with floaters
Yellow/white areas are seen on the retina, with
  areas of haemorrhage ('eggs and bacon').
  Retinal detachment sometimes occurs.
  Treatment is with ganciclovir. Differential
  diagnosis includes HIV, HSV, VZV and
  Toxoplasma

TREATMENT

Highly active antiretroviral therapy (HAART) is
the mainstay of treatment at present, typically
involving two reverse transcriptase inhibitors

plus a protease inhibitor. This can substantially delay the onset of the AIDS complex, delay death and reduce viral load to undetectable levels in many patients.

Important side effects include (vary between drugs)
Pancreatitis: ddI, lamivudine
Neuropathy: ddC, ddI, ritonavir
Anaemia and granulocytopenia:
    zidovudine
Myositis: zidovudine
Ulcers: ddC
Rash: nevirapine
Deranged LFTs: ritonavir
GI upset: protease inhibitors

PROGNOSIS

Improving. The average time from an AIDS defining illness to death is now well over 3 years. 25% of patients are predicted to live for more than 15 years from the time of infection.

QUESTION SPOTTING

Grey case
The presenting problem is likely to be an AIDS defining illness, e.g. *Pneumocystis* infection. A less likely scenario would be a patient known to be HIV positive developing a symptom complex, e.g. meningitis, or the presentation of a seroconversion illness.

Look for risk factors
Promiscuity
Haemophilia (may have a prolonged APTT)
Previous blood transfusions
Presence of hepatitis B or C (i.e. viruses
    transmitted in the same way)
Businessman, especially if a history of foreign
    travel
African or Asian travel

Also remember to look for other HIV related conditions when you have identified the major problem.

Data interpretation
Less likely to crop up in this section.

GONORRHOEA

Infection with *Neisseria gonorrhoeae*, a gram negative diplococcus, is almost always spread by sexual contact, and can colonize and infect the genitourinary tract, anus, rectum, pharynx and conjunctivae. Systemic infection occurs in less than 1% of cases.

FEATURES

Males
5% are asymptomatic
Dysuria
Urethral discharge
Rectal discharge

Females
More often asymptomatic
Cervical discharge (40%)
Dysuria (12%)

Other features
Epididymo-orchitis (2%)
Prostatitis, seminal vesiculitis
Periurethral abscesses
Endometritis
Salpingitis
Meningitis – rare

Fitz-Hugh Curtis syndrome (Perihepatitis)
RUQ pain
Shoulder tip pain
Fever
Tender hepatomegaly
Hepatic rub
Right-sided pleural effusion

Septicaemia (dermatitis/arthritis syndrome)
Large joint polyarthritis. Effusions may be present. Septic monoarthritis may occur
Tenosynovitis
Fever
Rash: maculopapular at first, becoming pustular, then haemorrhagic, and finally necrotic

INVESTIGATIONS

FBC
Hb normal
WCC may be ↑
Platelets normal

U + Es
Normal

LFTs
Elevated in septicaemia or perihepatitis
ESR may be elevated
ECG normal
CXR shows small right-sided effusion (Fitz-Hugh Curtis syndrome)
Joint X-ray usually normal
Joint fluid straw coloured or purulent

DIAGNOSIS

Culture; urethral swab in men, endocervical swab in women

Disseminated infection
Blood culture (25–75% sensitivity)
Joint aspirate (25–75% sensitivity)
Skin lesions (5–10% sensitivity)

DIFFERENTIAL DIAGNOSIS

Disseminated infection
Meningococcal septicaemia
Lyme disease
Secondary syphilis
SBE
Vasculitis

Fitz-Hugh Curtis syndrome
Chlamydia infection
Viral hepatitis
Right basal pneumonia

Urethritis
Chlamydia infection
Non-specific urethritis
Foreign body in urethra

TREATMENT

Simple infection
If organism is penicillin sensitive in population, use penicillin + probenecid (single dose).
Otherwise, use ciprofloxacin or ceftriaxone single dose. Chlamydia often co-infects, and should be eradicated (e.g. 1 week of doxycycline)

Disseminated infection
Parenteral cephalosporins for 48 h, then oral cephalosporin for 1 week
Test for other STDs

Trace sexual contacts

Test for cure at 4 and 10 days post-antibiotics; cure rate is very high

QUESTION SPOTTING

Grey cases

Will tend to present as either Fitz-Hugh Curtis syndrome or arthritis/dermatitis syndrome

Clues to the presence of an STD (in the examination) are:

A businessman

A history of a new relationship

Recent foreign travel or holiday

Data interpretation

Unlikely to crop up in this section.

LYME DISEASE

Infection by *Borrelia burgdorferi*, a spirochaete transmitted by ticks of the *Ixodes* genus. Rodents are the main reservoir for infection; some birds are also infected. Disease appears to be more virulent in the USA than in Europe; in particular, arthritis is very uncommon in European infection. Infection tends to peak around June to October.

FEATURES

Symptomless in up to 90%

Immediate (stage I)
Erythema migrans (90%): rash slowly (over weeks) spreads outwards from tick bite; centre may then clear. Multifocal rashes may occur.

Fever
Flu-like illness
Headache
Arthralgia
Regional lymphadenopathy

Delayed (stage II) (weeks)

Carditis (10%)
AV block
Myocarditis
Pericarditis

Neurological features (10–20%)
Meningitis
Cranial nerve palsies; especially VII nerve; may be bilateral
Radiculopathy
Encephalopathy
Peripheral neuropathy

Borrelia lymphocytoma: bluish nodule on nipple or ear

Chronic (stage III) (months to years)
Acrodermatitis chronica atrophicans (Europe only)
Migratory large joint oligoarthritis, especially in knees; often swollen but not hot or painful
Chronic neurological problems –
Polyneuropathy, cerebral vasculitis

Other features
Conjunctivitis occurs uncommonly (<5%)
Gastrointestinal and pulmonary involvement is extremely uncommon

INVESTIGATIONS

FBC
Usually normal

U + Es
Normal
LFTs
Mild ↑ of AST and ALT
ESR normal or ↑
Normal glucose
CSF shows pleocytosis
Synovial fluid shows moderately high WCC, mildly elevated protein

ECG
May show ST elevation (pericarditis)
T wave changes (myocarditis)
Long PR interval or higher grade AV block

DIAGNOSIS

Culture in patients presenting with rash; 100% specific and 55–85% sensitive
Culture in patients without rash; CSF, blood, urine and joint fluid all have a very poor yield
Serology: rising titres are unreliable particularly in populations where Lyme disease is endemic, e.g. forestry workers. Antibodies persist for years. False positives occur in a number of other diseases, including ehrlichiosis and babesiosis. Seroconversion takes up to 6 weeks. However, negative antibody tests are rare in chronic disease.

NB. Some features of Lyme disease may be due to co-infection with *Ehrlichia* or *Babesia* species; this is an area of some controversy at present.

DIFFERENTIAL DIAGNOSIS

Viral infections: pericarditis, encephalitis, meningitis, arthritis
Sarcoidosis especially bilateral VIIn palsy
Syphilis
Ehrlichiosis
Babesiosis
Lymphoma
Vasculitides
Reiter's disease and reactive arthritis

TREATMENT

For mild disease oral penicillins or
  tetracyclines
For cardiac or neurological disease IV
  ceftriaxone or IV penicillin

PROGNOSIS

Usually excellent once treated. Cardiac problems
usually resolve, but mild neurological deficit
may remain.

QUESTION SPOTTING

Grey case
Clues to the diagnosis are:

Bitten by a tick, or visited a known endemic area
Typical rash (too much of a giveaway in MRCP!)
AV block in a young or middle aged patient
Bilateral VIIn palsy, or VIIn palsy with arthritic
  symptoms
Indolent meningitis/encephalitis

Data interpretation
Unlikely to crop up in this section.

MALARIA

Caused by the parasite *Plasmodium*, of which there are four species: *vivax, ovale, falciparum* and *malariae*. Infection occurs following introduction of sporozoites via the female *Anopheles* mosquito.

The parasite life cycle length depends on the species: 48 h for *P. falciparum*, 48–72 h for *P. vivax* and *P. ovale*, and 72 h for *P. malariae*.

The different species also tend to have different capacities to infect the red cell. *P. falciparum* will infect any red cell, especially young ones and therefore tends to have the most severe effects. *P. vivax* and *P. ovale* tend to infect reticulocytes and immature red cells. *P. malariae* infects senescent red cells.

Patients with sickle cell disease, beta-thalassaemia, phosphate kinase deficiency, glucose-6-phosphate deficiency or Duffy negative red cells show resistance to malaria infection.

Incubation period of 10–14 days except for *P. malariae* (18 days to 6 weeks) which may be modified if anti-malarial chemoprophylaxis is used so that the clinical disease may not present for months after infection.

SYMPTOMS

Fever up to 41°C
Headache
Myalgia
Shortness of breath due to anaemia and/or
    metabolic acidosis
Confusion
Coma
Convulsions
Chest pain
Abdominal pain
Diarrhoea

SIGNS

Hepatomegaly
Splenomegaly
Meningism
Dysconjugate gaze
Extensor plantars
Hypotension

INVESTIGATIONS

FBC
Hb ↓
WCC ↑ (neutrophilia), normal or sometimes ↓
Platelets normal or ↓

U + Es
Na normal or often ↓
K normal
Urea and creatinine ↑ if renal failure

LFTs
ALP ↑
ALT ↑
Bilirubin ↑
Albumin ↓

Clotting
Prolonged clotting times if DIC

ESR ↑
CRP ↑

Haptoglobins ↓
Reticulocytes ↑

Urinalysis
Blood and protein if glomerulonephritis or acute
    tubular necrosis

DIAGNOSIS

Thick and thin blood films stained with Giemsa stain. *P. falciparum* only shows ring forms in the early stages, whereas the other species show all stages of the erythrocytic cycle. Multiple infection of a single erythrocyte suggests *falciparum*. 3–4 stains over a period of days may be required. Diagnosis may be difficult if the patient has been partially treated.

Serological blood tests are available that may be used in conjunction with blood films.

ASSOCIATIONS

Anaemia due to:

Haemolysis (both of infected and non-infected
    red cells)
Dyserythropoiesis
Sequestration secondary to splenomegaly
Folate deficiency

Herpes simplex

COMPLICATIONS

Glomerulonephritis and nephrotic syndrome seen in children, especially with *P. malariae* and this may be fatal.

Acute tubular necrosis with oliguria, uraemia and haemoglobinuria (black water fever).

Metabolic acidosis, septic shock.

Splenic rupture.

Cerebral oedema.

TREATMENT

Antipyretics such as paracetamol and salicylates. Fluids if dehydrated or shocked.

Exchange transfusion if heavy parasitaemia.

Phenobarbitone may be used to prevent fitting.

Specific treatment for acute attacks

Consult BNF or Tropical Diseases Centre for most up to date information. Currently:

P. vivax, P. ovale and *P. malariae*

Chloroquine 600 mg of the base, then 300 mg 6 h later, and then 150 mg twice daily for 3 days.

P. falciparum

Widespread resistance to chloroquine so treatment is quinine for 5–7 days followed by three tablets of pyrimethamine and sulfadoxine (Fansidar) as a stat dose.

An alternative is mefloquine. Resistance to mefloquine is now emerging. Halofantrine can also be used.

Eradication of liver forms

Essential for *P. vivax* and *P. ovale* which may re-present at a later date unless eradicated with primaquine.

Prevention

Passive prevention of mosquito bites is strongly recommended with repellents, mosquito nets and clothing to cover exposed skin.

Chloroquine in area of low resistance. Chloroquine and proguanil or mefloquine if resistance high. Mefloquine is contraindicated in first trimester of pregnancy, lactation, epilepsy, cardiac conduction disorders and psychiatric disorders.

DIFFERENTIAL DIAGNOSIS

Fevers

Pneumonia

Ascending cholangitis

Pyelonephritis

Hepatitis

Infective endocarditis

Infectious mononucleosis

Splenomegaly

Visceral leishmaniasis

Schistosomiasis

Tuberculosis

Brucellosis

Typhoid

Haematological and inflammatory causes

QUESTION SPOTTING

Grey case

More likely to be seen in this type of question. There should be a lead such as splenomegaly or a history of travel. This may not necessarily be recent, and the patient may well have taken the appropriate prophylaxis. Malaria is important to consider and exclude with thick and thin blood films. Also consider if fever is culture negative and does not respond to antibiotics.

Data interpretation

Less likely to occur in the setting.

TOXIC SHOCK SYNDROME

Localized infection, usually by *Staphylococcus aureus*, producing an exotoxin which causes widespread cytotoxic effects on multiple organ systems. TSS toxin 1 (TSST 1) is the toxin responsible in 75% of cases. Similar syndromes have been reported with *Staph. epidermidis* and streptococci as causative organisms. Two-thirds of cases are caused by infected tampons.

SYMPTOMS

Fever
Myalgia
Vomiting and diarrhoea
Confusion and drowsiness

The local source of infection may be from tampons, conjunctivitis, abscesses or burns.

SIGNS

Fever
Low BP, tachycardia
Macular rash, progressing to desquamation
May have tender muscles
May have a reduced conscious level
Vaginal discharge

INVESTIGATIONS

FBC
Hb usually normal
WCC often ↑
Platelets may be ↓

U + Es
Na usually normal
K may be ↑
Urea and creatinine ↑ in renal failure

LFTs
May be ↑
Calcium may be low
CK often raised
Clotting usually normal, but DIC can
    occur
Blood cultures almost always negative
CSF virtually never shows growth

DIAGNOSIS

Firm diagnosis is based on all five of:

1. Temperature >39°C
2. Macular rash
3. Systolic BP <90, or diastolic postural drop
4. Source of localized TSST producing infection
5. **Evidence of toxic action on 3 systems:**
    Diarrhoea/vomiting
    Myalgia/raised CK
    Drowsiness/confusion
    Raised urea/creatinine
    Reduced platelets

DIFFERENTIAL DIAGNOSIS

Septicaemic shock
Weil's disease
Measles
Rickettsial infections
Malaria

TREATMENT

Remove source of infection (tampon, abscess)
IV flucloxacillin
Supportive therapy for shock and renal failure.
    Shock is often resistant to fluid replacement
    and necessitates use of inotropic/vasopressor
    support

PROGNOSIS

10% mortality

QUESTION SPOTTING

Grey case

If you are lucky, there will be clues, e.g. tampon use, conjunctivitis or abscesses. If there are no clues, suspect the diagnosis in a young woman with a septic shock/multiorgan failure picture with no apparent cause.

Data interpretation

Likely to present in a similar way; suspect if a number of unrelated biochemical and haematological derangements appear in a young woman with fever of no obvious cause.

LEPTOSPIROSIS (WEIL'S DISEASE)

Infection with the spirochaete *Leptospira interrogans*. This is harboured by a wide variety of animals, but rats are the most common source of human infection. Severe disease involving hepatic and renal failure is known as Weil's disease. Anyone exposed to contaminated water or handling infected animals is at risk of infection; the organism can enter via broken skin or mucous membranes. The incubation period is 2 to 20 days. At risk groups include farmworkers, sewer workers, vets and watersports participants.

NB. Only 10–15% of infections result in severe liver and renal disease.

PHASE 1: infection (lasts 4 to 7 days)

Symptoms
Fever and chills (>85%)
Headache (>85%)
Myalgia (>85%)
Abdominal pain
Vomiting, diarrhoea
Delirium, hallucinations, psychosis
Arthralgia
Cough, sore throat, haemoptysis

Signs
Fever
Tachycardia
Hypotension
Splenomegaly (15–25%)
Hepatomegaly
Lymphadenopathy (15%)
Lung crackles
Meningism
Skin rash: purpuric, urticarial or maculopapular
Conjunctival suffusion

PHASE 2: immune response (lasts 4 to 30 days)

Symptoms
Headache, photophobia, neck stiffness (50–90%)
Sore eyes
Fever
Skin rash
Jaundice

Signs
Jaundice
Meningism
Reduced conscious level

Cranial nerve palsies, radiculopathy, focal weakness, fits and nystagmus may all occur
Hepatomegaly
Uveitis

INVESTIGATIONS

FBC
Hb often ↓ (haemolysis, bleeding)
WCC usually ↑
Platelets may be ↓

U + Es
Urea and creatinine often ↑ (65%)

LFTs
Bilirubin may be very ↑
ALT slightly ↑
ALP ↑
Reticulocytes may be ↑
Haptoglobins may be ↓
ESR ↑
LDH ↑
CK may be ↑
PO_4 ↑ if renal impairment severe
Urate ↑ if renal impairment severe
Clotting abnormal (liver disease or DIC)
D-dimers ↑ (in DIC)
Blood film may show fragmented RBCs and polychromasia
Urine proteinuria (usually <1 g/24 h). Microscopic haematuria and leucocytes
CSF pleocytosis. Glucose normal, protein slightly raised

DIAGNOSIS

Blood cultures and CSF may grow organisms on days 0 to 10 of illness
Urine culture may be positive from 2nd to 4th week
Serology (agglutination testing): positive from week 2. Titres of >1 : 100 are diagnostic
PCR testing for Weil's disease is also now available

DIFFERENTIAL DIAGNOSIS

Other haemorrhagic fevers (e.g. Dengue)
Yellow fever
Viral hepatitis

EBV infection
Brucellosis
Atypical pneumonias
Malaria
Aseptic meningitis
Relapsing fever
Hepatorenal syndrome
Paracetamol overdose
CCl_4 toxicity
Amanita phalloides poisoning
Toxaemia of pregnancy
HUS/TTP
Incompatible blood transfusion

COMPLICATIONS

Liver failure
Acute renal failure
DIC, microangiopathic anaemia
ARDS
Cardiac arrhythmias
Jarisch-Herxheimer reaction on starting
   antibiotics

TREATMENT

Support for vital organs
IV penicillin or tetracyclines

Prophylactic antibiotics may avoid infection if
given after exposure to water known to be
infected.

PROGNOSIS

Good recovery in most cases; renal function
usually recovers fully. Between 5 and 20%
mortality seen in patients with full blown Weil's
disease.

QUESTION SPOTTING

Grey case
Clues to the diagnosis are:
Exposure to rodents, sewers or watersports
A job as a vet or farmworker
Presence of meningism
Combined hepatic and renal dysfunction
Myalgia and conjunctival suffusion as a
   prominent symptom
A biphasic illness (may be asymptomatic for
   1 to 3 days between infectious and immune
   phases)

Data interpretation
Less likely to crop up in this section, but again,
look out for combined hepatic and renal failure
in a patient with exposure risk factors.

BOTULISM

Ingestion of a 150 kD, heat stable toxin produced by *Clostridium botulinum*. Ingestion of the bacterium itself is unnecessary. The most common source is canned foods which have not been adequately heat treated (spores are heat resistant and require temperatures of up to 120°C to ensure eradication)

Botulinum toxin is absorbed via mucous membranes, and spreads haematogenously to neuromuscular junctions, where it inhibits cholinergic transmission irreversibly. Recovery therefore requires new motor end-plate formation.

SYMPTOMS

Onset 2–48 h after ingestion:
Nausea, vomiting
Double vision
Blurred vision
Dry mouth
Constipation
Urinary retention
Muscle weakness
Difficulty breathing
Dysarthria

SIGNS

Conscious level preserved
Descending paralysis; cranial nerves affected first
Convergent strabismus
Fixed mid range or dilated pupils
Ptosis
Reduced tone and power
Reflexes preserved at first
Labile BP; may be low

Note that fever is unusual.

INVESTIGATIONS

FBC
Usually normal

U + Es
Usually normal

LFTs
Usually normal

ECG may show non-specific ST/T abnormalities
Nerve conduction studies normal
EMG shows reduced amplitude discharges, but may increase after tetanic stimulation

PFTs
FVC may drop quickly
FEV1 drops in parallel

Anti-AChR antibodies negative
Anti-calcium channel antibodies negative
CSF protein may be slightly elevated. No increase in cell numbers
Tensilon test may be weakly positive

DIAGNOSIS

Demonstration of toxin in faeces, blood or food by mouse bioassay.

DIFFERENTIAL DIAGNOSIS

Guillain-Barré syndrome (especially Miller-Fisher variant)
Myasthenia gravis
Poliomyelitis
Tick paralysis
Familial periodic paralysis
Drug induced neuromuscular block
Shellfish poisoning

TREATMENT

Deaths usually occur from respiratory paralysis, thus close monitoring of the FVC and mechanical respiratory support is crucial. Antitoxin against A, B and E toxins (those usually responsible) probably reduces death rates. Some centres also give penicillin to clear any clostridia which may have colonized the gut.

Respiratory support may have to be given for between 30 and 100 days; ventilator failure, tracheostomy complications and infection may supervene.

PROGNOSIS

Mortality in the UK with appropriate support is currently 10% or less.

QUESTION SPOTTING

Grey case

Clues in the grey case are:
Descending paralysis
No sensory involvement
No impairment of consciousness
Afebrile

The tensilon test is usually normal (excluding myasthenia), and the CSF protein is not greatly raised (in contrast with Guillain-Barré syndrome).

Data interpretation

Unlikely to crop up, but possible as an abbreviated version of the above, with tensilon test and CSF results.

HAEMATOLOGY

HYPOGAMMAGLOBULINAEMIA

Subclassification
Primary
X-linked agammaglobulinaemia
Common variable immunodeficiency (CVID)
Selective IgG subclass deficiency
IgA deficiency
Thymoma with hypogammaglobulinaemia
Transient infantile hypogammaglobulinaemia
Transcobalamin II deficiency

Secondary
Chronic lymphocytic leukaemia
Myeloma
Protein losing enteropathy
Nephrotic syndrome
Myotonic dystrophy
Drugs; gold, phenytoin, penicillamine (the latter
    two usually IgA selective)

X-linked (Bruton's) agammaglobulinaemia
This disease is rare. Patients usually start to
develop infections once the maternal IgG
disappears from the stream blood at 3 months
onwards. IgG levels are detectable but are
<50 mg/100 ml. T cells are present in normal
numbers and function normally, but there are no
mature B cells.

Common variable immunodeficiency
Onset at any age, but peak incidence is in the
    third decade. There is no HLA matching.
    There is a slight increase in incidence of
    selective IgA deficiency in relatives.
IgA is often virtually absent. IgG levels vary but
    are usually <200 mg/100 ml. IgM may be low
    or even raised.
30% have lymphopenia and associated
    splenomegaly.
T cells are often functionally immature as may
    be the macrophages. There may therefore be a
    reduced level of cellular immunity, but the
    infections associated with T cell deficiencies
    are rare.

Selective IgG subclass deficiency
May be either inherited or acquired. The most
common type is the IgG2 subclass which is
involved in immunity to polysaccharides and
deficiency has been associated with poor
response to polysaccharide vaccines and an
increase in certain pulmonary infections.

However most patients have normal lives and life
expectancy.

Selective IgA subclass deficiency
Very common with an incidence of 1 : 700 in
Caucasians. The disease is usually sporadic but
may be inherited as a defect in chromosome 18.
Associations include ataxia telangiectasia;
coeliac disease (may be due to the common
association with HLA DR3 but may be directly
due to the deficiency itself), rheumatoid
arthritis, Still's disease and epilepsy, due
to the use of gold, penicillamine and
phenytoin.
   It is important to check for IgA deficiency
prior to truncal vagotomy as this reduces gut
motility and causes bacterial overgrowth in these
patients leading to chronic diarrhoea and
malabsorption.
   Patients with IgA deficiency should be tested
for IgA auto antibodies (the presence of which is
a contraindication to blood transfusion or
gammaglobulin treatment as this can cause
anaphylaxis unless depleted of IgA).

Most common pathogens
Streptococcus – pneumonia, meningitis, septic
    arthritis
Haemophilus influenzae – pneumonia,
    meningitis, septic arthritis
Staphylococcus – pyoderma and septic arthritis
    (esp. children)
Mycoplasma pneumoniae – pneumonia and
    arthritis
Campylobacter – gastrointestinal infection
Giardia – gastrointestinal infection
Ureaplasma urealyticum – chronic urinary tract
    infection
Herpes zoster – shingles
Enteroviruses – diarrhoea, chronic meningitis
    and myositis

SYMPTOMS
Vary according to infective organism.
Watch for symptoms of meningism, septic
    arthritis, pneumonia, infective diarrhoea,
    urinary tract infections, shingles and
    myositis.
No symptoms directly due to
    hypogammaglobulinaemia.

SIGNS

Lymphadenopathy
Pulmonary crackles from chest infections,
   bronchiectasis and fibrosis
Splenomegaly associated with nodular lymphoid
   hyperplasia

INVESTIGATIONS

FBC

Hb normal
WCC variable. May be ↑ in infection or ↓ if
   X-linked agammaglobulinaemia
Platelets normal

U + Es

Normal

LFTs

Normal
Rheumatoid factor negative
Urinary protein normal
Faecal ^{51}CR transferrin normal, cf. protein losing
   enteropathy

Synovial fluid

Mononuclear infiltrate
Positive culture if septic arthritis

DIAGNOSIS

Immunoglobulins ↓
Protein electrophoresis is normal or has ↓ γ band

DIFFERENTIAL DIAGNOSIS

Selective class hypogammaglobulinaemia
Lymphoma
Leukaemia
Rheumatoid arthritis including Felty's syndrome
Other causes of bronchiectasis, including cystic
   fibrosis

Other causes of chronic diarrhoea

COMPLICATIONS

Bronchiectasis
Pulmonary fibrosis
Cor pulmonale
Malabsorption
Gastric carcinoma ($\times$ 50 risk)
Non-erosive arthritis – symmetrical polyarthritis
   which usually spares hands and feet
Tenosynovitis
Achlorhydria (30%). Some of these lack intrinsic
   factor and develop pernicious anaemia
Autoimmune disease
Lymphoreticular malignancy

TREATMENT

Gammaglobulin – frequency and dose depends
   on the clinical experience of the patient
Antibiotics for acute infection
Physiotherapy for bronchiectasis
Antibiotic prophylaxis with low dose penicillin
   is advised

QUESTION SPOTTING

Grey case

Watch for recurrent infections and arthritis
especially if there is lymphadenopathy or
splenomegaly. If the albumin and the total
protein are given always work out the globulins
to exclude hypogammaglobulinaemia. Need to
exclude Felty's syndrome (↑↑ rheumatoid factor,
leucopenia, anaemia and thrombocytopenia.
Immunoglobulins raised).

Data interpretation

Unlikely to appear in this section.

PAROXYSMAL NOCTURNAL HAEMOGLOBINURIA

An acquired clonal abnormality of bone marrow stem cells, thought to produce deficiency of glucosylphosphatidylinositol (GPI) in cell membranes. This lipid acts as an anchor for several membrane proteins, including those which protect cells against complement mediated lysis. Thus red cell, white cell and platelet lines become hypersensitive to complement lysis and are therefore reduced in number. The disease usually affects those between 20 and 40 years of age.

Haemolysis is mostly intravascular, and the remaining platelets can be activated inappropriately, leading to thrombotic complications.

SYMPTOMS

Tiredness
Shortness of breath
Dark urine due to haemoglobinuria. This is classically worse overnight, but may occur at any time
Headache
Abdominal pain

SIGNS

Jaundice (usually mild)
Splenomegaly
Hepatomegaly
Purpura (if severe)

INVESTIGATIONS

FBC
Hb ↓
MCV slightly ↑
Reticulocytes ↑
WCC ↓
Neutrophil ALP score ↓
Platelets ↓

U + Es
Usually normal

LFTs
Bilirubin ↑ (unconjugated, so not found in urine)
Fe often ↓
TIBC often ↑
Haptoglobins absent

Marrow biopsy shows hypoplastic marrow in many cases. Low iron stores
Urine shows haemoglobin in urine.
Haemosiderin is also detectable in urine (derived from tubular cells taking up haem pigment from circulation)

DIAGNOSIS

Ham's test: ABO compatible serum, acidified to pH 6.5 is incubated with the red cells for 60 min. A proportion (not all) of the cells are lysed in PNH, whereas none are lysed in a normal sample. Note that osmotic fragility is normal in PNH.

ASSOCIATIONS

Aplastic anaemia (this precedes PNH in 25%)
Myelofibrosis
Acute myeloblastic leukaemia (rare)

COMPLICATIONS

Thrombotic disease, usually venous. There is a predilection to portal vein thrombosis and Budd-Chiari syndrome, as well as DVT and PE.
Pigment gallstones (secondary to longstanding haemolysis).
Bacterial infections (due to granulocytopenia).

TREATMENT

Bone marrow transplant if disease is severe, otherwise supportive treatment with blood transfusion, iron supplements (secondary iron deficiency is common due to loss of haemoglobin in the urine). Venous thrombosis necessitates therapy with warfarin, but prophylaxis is not used. Steroids have no effect on the course or severity of the disease.

PROGNOSIS

7.5 year median survival, but 10–15% remit spontaneously

QUESTION SPOTTING

Grey case

Think of PNH when:
Venous thromboemboli occur, especially in conjunction with pancytopenia.
Whenever there is a past history of aplastic anaemia.

The history of haemoglobinuria is often long, unlike other causes of haemolysis listed below.

Data interpretation

Look for a haemolytic picture with haemoglobinuria and pancytopenia.
The differential diagnosis for data interpretation includes:

DIC
HUS/TTP
CLL and other reticuloendothelial malignancy

VITAMIN B₁₂ DEFICIENCY

Vitamin B_{12} is absorbed in the terminal ileum, and body stores may last between 3–5 years in the absence of dietary B_{12}. Deficiency chiefly affects haematopoietic cell turnover and neural tissues. The mechanism of neuronal dysfunction is unclear; the effect on bone marrow is due to defective DNA synthesis.

Causes
Dietary (e.g. vegans)

Lack of intrinsic factor
Pernicious anaemia
Gastrectomy
Gastric carcinoma

Small bowel dysfunction
Bacterial overgrowth
Crohn's disease
Ileal resection
Fish tapeworm
HIV infection
Tropical sprue
Radiation enteritis

Transcobalamin II deficiency

SYMPTOMS

Sore tongue (glossitis)
Diarrhoea (intestinal dysfunction)
Indigestion
Weight loss
Tiredness, SOB
Easy bruising
Numbness and tingling in limbs
Unsteadiness, limb weakness
Memory loss
Visual loss

SIGNS

General
Pale
Bruising occasionally seen
Red, shiny tongue
Skin pigmentation (occasional)
Pyrexia (up to 38°C)
Splenomègaly (mild)

Neurological
Optic atrophy

Altered sensation in limbs
Limb weakness
Reduced ankle reflexes
Extensor plantars
Loss of vibration and joint position sense

INVESTIGATIONS

FBC
Hb ↓
MCV markedly ↑
Reticulocytes ↓
WCC often ↓
Platelets often ↓

U + Es
Normal

LFTs
Bilirubin may be ↑ (haemolysis)
ALT mildly ↑
ALP ↓

Clotting normal
Ferritin ↑
Fe ↑
LDH elevated (haemolysis)
Haptoglobins low or absent
Cholesterol low

Blood film
Macrocytic RBCs
Hypersegmented (>5) neutrophils

Bone marrow:

Megaloblasts
Giant metamyelocytes

DIAGNOSIS

B₁₂ deficiency
Low serum B_{12} with normal or low folate

Pernicious anaemia
Parietal cell antibodies are positive in 90% of cases. Intrinsic Factor (IF) antibodies are present in 50% and are specific for pernicious anaemia.

To differentiate lack of intrinsic factor from small bowel disease
Schilling test:

1 mcg of radiolabelled B$_{12}$ is given orally
1 mg of unlabelled B$_{12}$ is then given IM to
    saturate the body stores and mobilize the oral
    dose
Urine is collected for 24 h
Normal subjects should excrete >10% of the
    radioactive dose

If the test is abnormal, IF is given orally with the
radiolabelled B$_{12}$. If the test corrects to normal,
lack of IF (i.e. a gastric problem) is to blame.

DIFFERENTIAL DIAGNOSIS

Usually of other causes of megaloblastic
anaemia, most commonly folate deficiency,
which may coexist.

TREATMENT

Intramuscular B$_{12}$ injections. Haematological
response is evident within a few days;
neurological symptoms may reverse entirely over
a few months provided B$_{12}$ deficiency is not
longstanding.

ASSOCIATIONS

Associations with pernicious anaemia:
IDDM
Addison's disease
Vitiligo
Hypothyroidism
Graves' disease
Primary ovarian failure
Hypoparathyroidism
IgA deficiency
Hypogammaglobulinaemia
Gastric carcinoma
Lambert-Eaton syndrome
Myasthenia gravis

QUESTION SPOTTING

Grey case

May occur as part of a grey case; pernicious
anaemia is perhaps less likely than one of the
small intestinal causes. Note that B$_{12}$ deficiency
is one of the causes of absent ankle reflexes plus
extensor plantars.

   Look out for anaemia or pancytopenia plus
neurological signs, perhaps complicating a case
of Crohn's disease or several years after
radiotherapy for cervical cancer.

Data interpretation

Usually relies on interpretation of the Schilling
test. Beware incongruous or nonsensical results
on the Schilling test; it usually means that the
24 h urine collection is incomplete.

MYELODYSPLASIA

Generally thought of as a group of preleukaemic disorders, with neoplastic change and ineffective haematopoiesis. There are abnormalities of peripheral blood and bone marrow function, which may eventually evolve into an acute myeloid leukaemia.

Although there are many classifications, the simplest is primary (no known cause), and secondary, as a result of treatment with alkylating agents with or without radiotherapy for the treatment of myeloma, lymphoma and other cancers. The FAB classification is widely used and recognized, and can be seen in Table 1.

The patient is usually over 50 years of age (the peak incidence is in the seventies) and men and women are equally affected.

SYMPTOMS

May be asymptomatic
Tiredness
Shortness of breath
Easy bruising, excessive bleeding
Recurrent infections
Fever

SIGNS

Anaemia
Bruising
Splenomegaly (10–20%)

INVESTIGATIONS

FBC
Hb ↓
MCV ↑ or normal

WCC ↓ or ↑
Platelets ↓ but may be normal
Reticulocytes ↓

U&Es
Normal

LFTs
Normal
Blood film – anisopoikylocytosis, polychromasia, punctate basophilia, abnormal neutrophils, and blasts may be present. Giant platelets may be seen.

DIAGNOSIS

Bone marrow aspiration
Erythroid lineage: abnormal nuclear shape with nuclear fragments, and ring sideroblasts.
Myeloid lineage: ↓ granules in neutrophils and myelocytes. Hyposegmented (Pelger cells) or hypersegmented neutrophils. Blasts.
Megakaryocytic lineage: micromegakaryocytes, megakaryocytes with abnormal nuclei.

Bone marrow trephine
Shows hypercellularity with little or no fat space. Clusters of blasts can be seen. Fibrosis is not a feature of primary myelodysplasia, but may be seen in secondary.

DIFFERENTIAL DIAGNOSIS

Anaemia secondary to folate/vitamin B_{12} deficiency
Anaemia secondary to chronic diseases such as liver/renal disease or chronic inflammation.
Overt leukaemias such as AML.

Table 1   FAB classification of myelodysplasia

Type	Peripheral blood		Bone marrow
Refractory anaemia (RA)	<1% blasts	and	<5% blasts
Refractory anaemia with ring sideroblasts (RARS)	<1% blasts	and	<5% blasts, >15% sideroblasts
Refractory anaemia with excess blasts (RAEB)	<5% blasts	and	5–20% blasts
Refractory anaemia with excess blasts in transformation (RAEBt)	>5% blasts	and	21–30% blasts
Chronic myelomonocytic leukaemia (CMML)	$>1.0 \times 10^9$/L monocytes	and	<30% blasts puls promonocytes

TREATMENT

Supportive therapy with red cell and platelet
  transfusions.
Antibiotic therapy for infection.
Chemotherapy if fit and motivated and younger
  patients with more severe disease, but
  long-term outcomes are still poor. Low dose
  hydroxyurea or etoposide can improve white
  counts and spleen size but, again, long-term
  outlook is poor.
Bone marrow transplantation is the only curative
  therapy but only 40–60% are disease free after
  5 years.

PROGNOSIS

Highly variable. Median survival is about
  20 months.

One-third die of unrelated conditions.
One-third die of leukaemic
  transformation.
One-third die of marrow failure without
  transformation.

QUESTION SPOTTING

Grey case

The typical patient will be in their 60–80s and
will present with symptoms of anaemia,
infection or bruising. Diagnosis comes from
bone marrow examination.

Data interpretation

You may be asked to interpret a bone marrow or
blood film. Pelger cells should alert you to this
diagnosis.

SICKLE CELL DISEASE

Hereditary disorder of haemoglobin structure where valine has been substituted for glutamic acid at position 6 of the haem β chain, caused by a point mutation. The abnormal HbS is insoluble in the deoxygenized form so polymerizes, and makes the red blood cell inflexible and take up the classic sickle shape. This is initially reversible, but after repeated sickling episodes, the cell becomes fixed in the sickled shape. The sickled red blood cells have a shortened life span due to increased fragility, and this leads to a chronic haemolytic anaemia. The cells can aggregate, increasing blood viscosity and cause arterial occlusion and tissue infarction. Sickling is precipitated by hypoxia, acidosis, infection, dehydration and cold. Many crisis episodes have no obvious precipitant.

The disease is common in but not exclusive to peoples of Equatorial African ancestry. Sickle disease is caused by inheriting abnormal haemoglobin genes from both parents. The most common cause of this is SS disease. However other abnormalities such as HbC, and the β-thalassaemias can occur in conjunction with HbS to give HbSC disease which has a similar course to HbSS disease, but with a slightly increased risk of thrombosis, and sickle cell/thalassaemia disease. People with only one abnormal HbS gene have the sickle cell trait which gives a usually harmless carrier state which also gives some resistance to malaria.

The sickle cell gene occurs with a frequency of up to 30% in Africa, Southern Europe and some parts of India.

CLINICAL FEATURES

All clinical features arise from the two main features of the disease
Haemolysis
Vaso-occlusive disease

Haemolysis
Anaemia – though this is rarely symptomatic except during crisis, as HbS releases oxygen to the tissues more easily, and there is increased cardiac output.
Bone marrow enlargement may lead to frontal bossing.

Hyperdynamic circulation may lead to heart failure and cardiomegaly.
Gallstones common (pigment) (up to 40% of 20 year olds with sickle cell disease).
Haemolysis increased by certain drugs, infection, or in association with G6PD deficiency.
Aplastic anaemia can occur as a result of certain viral infections especially parvovirus B19.

Vaso-occlusive disease
Bone pain (70%) with dactylitis and avascular necrosis and impaired growth in children.
Acute chest syndrome (40%) – fever, cough, dyspnoea, and pleuritic pain caused by combinations of infection, infarction, pulmonary sequestration and fat embolism.
Leg ulcers (20%). Rare in HbSC disease.
Genito-urinary – priapism (10–40%), impotence.
Renal (5–20%) – infarcts causing haematuria, and renal tubular defects, chronic renal failure, enuresis.
Cerebral – strokes (10%) (commonest in childhood, and rare after 14 years of age), fits, and cognitive impairment.
Late puberty (average menarche 2.5 years late) may give rise to above average adult height.
Spleen – upper abdominal pain, acute enlargement (acute splenic sequestration), chronic enlargement (hypersplenism) and eventually splenic fibrosis (asplenia) leading to increased risk from capsulated bacteria, especially pneumococcus septicaemia, and *Salmonella* or *Staphylococcus aureus* osteomyelitis.
Liver (2%) – abnormal liver function tests with upper abdominal pain.
Watch out for secondary haemochromotosis from iron overload due to multiple transfusions.
Retinopathy – retinal detachment and proliferative retinopathy (rare in HbSS but up to 50% in HbSC).
Complications during pregnancy such as acute chest syndrome, and crisis (maternal mortality 1%). Spontaneous abortion common.

INVESTIGATIONS

FBC
Hb 6–9 g/dL steady state, but 3–4 g/dL during crisis

WCC normal

Platelets normal

Reticulocytes 5–15% steady state, 20–30% during crisis or low if aplastic crisis

U + Es

Na normal

K normal

Urea and creatinine ↑ if renal failure

LFTs

Bilirubin ↑

AST may be ↑

ALP may be ↑

Albumin may be ↓

Folate deficiency may give rise to megaloblastic anaemia with low reticulocyte counts, ↑ MCV and ↓ Hb

ABGs

pO_2 ↓

pCO_2 ↓

pH ↓

Chest X-ray

Infection

Infarction

Avascular necrosis of ribs

Infiltrates

Fibrosis

Bone X-rays to demonstrate avascular necrosis (esp. femoral heads)

Liver ultrasound may show gallstones

DIAGNOSIS

Blood film may show sickled cells and hyposplenism. Sickling can be induced by sodium metabisulphite.

Hb electrophoresis confirms diagnosis.

TREATMENT

Sickle crisis

Oxygen

Adequate pain relief, e.g. intravenous opiates

Vigorous rehydration

Broad spectrum antibiotics

Consider exchange transfusion (esp. if chest syndrome with hypoxia, stroke or priapism) to reduce HbS below 30%

Other management

Prophylactic penicillin for prevention of pneumococcal infection.

Aggressive management of blood pressure to prevent strokes.

Folate supplements in pregnancy.

Transfusion is only required on a regular basis if severe anaemia or frequent crises. Transfusions are often given prior to elective surgery and exchange transfusion may be needed before emergency surgery.

Splenectomy may be required for hypersplenism.

Hydroxyurea may be useful in adults, but long-term effects are unknown.

Bone marrow transplantation is still experimental. Hazards are high, and it is only indicated for patients under 16 years of age, with severe complications and an HLA matched donor (only about 1% of patients).

PROGNOSIS

Approximately 120 000 babies per year are born in Africa with sickle cell disease but <2% survive to 5 years old. Highest mortality is in the first year of life, especially the second 6 months when HbF levels have fallen. In industrialized nations, the prognosis is much better, and some patients survive to normal ages. However there is much variability from patient to patient.

QUESTION SPOTTING

Grey case

With the diverse complications of this disease, sickle cell disease is ideal for grey case questions. Think about it as a cause of abdominal pain, and gallstones. The nationality of the patient in the question may not be given.

Consider in any patient of Afro-Caribbean origin. Also consider in chest pain and shortness of breath in a young patient with anaemia.

Data interpretation

You may be asked to look at a full blood count result and asked to comment. The data may suggest a haemolytic anaemia, and sickle cell disease should be considered here.

MIXED ESSENTIAL CRYOGLOBULINAEMIA

Mixed cryoglobulinaemia is caused by immune complexes that precipitate at low temperatures (cryoglobulins). There are two components, a polyclonal IgG as antigen, and either a monoclonal IgM (Type II) or a polyclonal IgM (Type III), with anti IgG Fc specificity, i.e. rheumatoid factor activity.

Causes of mixed essential cryoglobulinaemia

Type II
Hepatitis C (90%)
Hepatitis B
SBE
EBV
CMV

Type III
Lyme disease
Syphilis
Coccidiomycosis
Malaria
SLE
Rheumatoid arthritis
Systemic sclerosis
Sjögren's syndrome

FEATURES

Lower limb purpura (95–100%)
Arthralgia (70–90%); NB. Arthritis is uncommon
Hepatitis; usually chronic (60–70%)
Sensorimotor peripheral neuropathy
    (20–70%)
Membranoproliferative glomerulonephritis
    (30–50%) leading to hypertension, nephrotic
    syndrome and renal impairment
Leg ulcers (30%)
Raynaud's syndrome (20%)
Abdominal pain (20%)
Sjögren's syndrome (15–40%)
Other features include hyperviscosity syndrome,
    pulmonary vasculitis and pleuropericarditis

INVESTIGATIONS

FBC
Hb may be $\downarrow$
WCC variable
Platelets variable

U + Es
Urea and creatinine may be $\uparrow$

LFTs
ALT, ALP often $\uparrow$
ESR raised
Igs may be $\downarrow$
Complement: low C1q, C2, C4 and total
    complement activity. Normal C3, C9

Autoantibodies
ANA positive in 5%
Antimitochondrial positive in 5%
Anti smooth muscle positive in 13%
Extractable nuclear antigens positive in 3%

DIAGNOSIS

Is on clinical grounds, together with the demonstration of cryoglobulins. Analysis of the cryoprecipitate then determines which category of cryoglobulinaemia is present.

DIFFERENTIAL DIAGNOSIS

Other vasculitides
SBE
Other causes of liver disease
Amyloidosis

COMPLICATIONS

Liver cirrhosis
B cell non-Hodgkin's lymphoma (5–10%)
Renal failure

TREATMENT

High dose steroids, with or without cytotoxics. Because 90% of cases are probably caused by hepatitis C infection, interferon alpha has been used with some effect.

QUESTION SPOTTING

Grey case
The triad of cutaneous vasculitis, renal involvement and arthralgia should raise the diagnosis. Other clues are:
Deranged LFTs
Risk factors for hepatitis C infection

Data interpretation
Less likely to crop up in this section.

THALASSAEMIAS

Abnormalities of haemoglobin synthesis which result in reduced output of one or other of the globin chains in adult haemoglobin. Each adult haemoglobin has four chains, two α and two β. Abnormalities of α chain production occur following mutations on the short arm of chromosome 16, while those of the β chain occur with mutations of chromosome 11. However the α chain genes are duplicated. Thalassaemias may arise from over 200 different mutations resulting in loss of α and β chain production either as a direct mutation of the globin chain or affecting translation or transcription processes.

Thalassaemias are common and are distributed across the Mediterranean region (especially beta-thalassaemia) the Middle East, the Indian subcontinent and South-East Asia (especially alpha-thalassaemia). It is not uncommon to see combinations of abnormalities such as thalassaemias and sickle cell to give sickle cell thalassaemias.

BETA-THALASSAEMIA SYNDROMES

The disease has a wide range of presentations and severities depending on whether there is no beta chain production ($\beta0$) or reduced production ($\beta+$). It also depends on whether the individual is homozygous or heterozygous for a defect or has more than one defect. The imbalance of α and β chains leads to precipitation of α chains causing ineffective erythropoiesis and haemolysis.

The syndromes tend to be divided into:

Thalassaemia major (Cooley's anaemia)
Thalassaemia intermedia
Thalassaemia trait or minor

Thalassaemia major

Clinical features
Severe anaemia
Splenomegaly
Hepatomegaly
Bony changes due to bone marrow expansion – so called 'hair on end' appearance and frontal bossing
Growth retardation
Failure to thrive
Recurrent infections

Thalassaemia intermedia

Tends to present with milder symptoms, and is often caused by mild $\beta+$ syndromes where beta chain production is mildly impaired or in combination with alpha-thalassaemia.

Patients present later with
Moderate anaemia (Hb 7–10 g/dL)
Splenomegaly
Bony deformities
Recurrent leg ulcers
Recurrent infections
Gallstones

Thalassaemia trait or minor

An asymptomatic condition. Patients may have mild anaemia or normal haemoglobin levels. However, they do have abnormalities on investigation such as microcytic (MCV 50–70 fl) hypochromic (MCH 20–22 pg) red cells (iron stores are normal) and often a raised Hb A2 and sometimes Hb F fractions.

INVESTIGATIONS

FBC
Hb ↓ (variable amount)
MCV and MCH ↓↓ – out of proportion to anaemia
WCC and platelets normal unless co-existent hypersplenism

U + Es
Normal

LFTs
Bilirubin ↑ if severe
TIBC may be saturated and ferritin high because repeated transfusions cause iron overload

Blood film
Hypochromia
Microcytosis
Nucleated red cells
Basophilic stippling
Target cells
Raised reticulocyte count

Diagnosis

Hb electrophoresis
Hb F ↑
Hb A2 ↑ or normal
Hb A ↓ or absent

Treatment

Transfusions to maintain Hb.

Iron chelation with desferrioxamine if necessary. Desferrioxamine is associated with ocular and acoustic nerve complications with long-term treatment and may lead to growth retardation and bone disease if given in large doses.

Folic acid therapy.

Splenectomy if hypersplenism.

Bone marrow transplantation should be considered in early life before iron overload or other complications occur.

Iron therapy is contraindicated.

Prognosis

50% patients die by the age of 35 years, often due to iron overload from repeated transfusions, and suboptimal iron chelation.

ALPHA-THALASSAEMIA SYNDROMES

Unlike the beta-thalassaemias, these all arise from gene deletions. As the alpha genes are duplicated, four scenarios may arise:

Single gene deletion ($-\alpha/\alpha\alpha$)

Asymptomatic carrier. Minority show $\downarrow$ MCV and MCH

Two gene deletions ($-\alpha/-\alpha$ or $--/\alpha\alpha$)

Alpha-thalassaemia trait – microcytosis with or without mild anaemia. Low MCV and MCH but asymptomatic.

Three gene deletions ($--/-\alpha$)

Hb H disease (Hb $\beta4$) – moderate haemolytic anaemia (Hb 7–10 g/dL) and splenomegaly, hepatomegaly, jaundice, leg ulcers, gallstones and folate deficiency. Hb H is seen in older red cells on blood film.

Four gene deletions ($--/--$)

Hb Barts (Hb $\gamma4$) – no α chain production. Hb $\gamma4$ is not able to carry oxygen, and infants are either stillborn at 28–40 weeks, or die soon after birth. They are pale, oedematous with huge spleens and livers – hydrops fetalis.

Treatment

Nil specific

Folic acid if necessary

Avoid iron therapy

QUESTION SPOTTING

Grey case

Could appear with sickle cell or alone. The key for thalassaemia is that the MCV and MCH are disproportionately low for the degree of anaemia. Also suspect this disease in Mediterranean/Arabic patients.

Data interpretation

Watch out for confusion with iron deficiency anaemia. Also note that Hb A2 may be falsely low with co-existing iron deficiency.

ANTIPHOSPHOLIPID SYNDROME (HUGHES SYNDROME)

Presence of an antibody which may either target phospholipids in cell membranes, or may react with β_2 glycoproteins bound to phospholipids in cell membranes. Antiphospholipid antibodies may be found in isolation (primary disease) or may accompany other autoimmune diseases, e.g. SLE.

CLINICAL FEATURES

Recurrent miscarriages

Venous thrombosis
DVT
PE
Pulmonary hypertension
Budd–Chiari syndrome
Dural sinus thrombosis

Arterial thrombosis
CVA/TIA
Mesenteric/peripheral thrombosis
MI
Endocarditis
Livedo reticularis

Less common features
Pyoderma gangrenosum
Acrocyanosis
Haemolytic anaemia
Transverse myelopathy

INVESTIGATIONS

FBC
Hb occasionally ↓
WCC normal
Platelets usually ↓

U + Es
Normal

LFTs
Normal unless syndrome is part of another disease.

INR normal
VDRL often positive
Anticardiolipin antibody often positive

DIAGNOSIS

Diagnostic criteria are one
Recurrent miscarriage
Arterial or venous thrombosis
Immune thrombocytopenia

plus

Anticardiolipin antibodies

or

Prolonged APTT or dilute Russell's viper venom test not correctible with normal plasma

ASSOCIATIONS

Autoimmune disease
Rheumatoid arthritis
SLE
Giant cell arteritis
Systemic sclerosis
Sjögren's syndrome
Psoriatic arthropathy

Infections, especially
Syphilis
Malaria
Hepatitis C
HIV

Drugs
Phenytoin
Hydralazine
Quinidine

Early, severe pre-eclampsia
IV drug abuse
Behçet's disease
Sickle cell anaemia
Guillain-Barré syndrome

DIFFERENTIAL DIAGNOSIS

Other causes of thrombophilia, including
Factor V Leiden mutation
Protein C deficiency
Protein S deficiency
Antithrombin III deficiency
Hyperhomocysteinaemia
Polycythaemia

ential thrombocythaemia
Paroxysmal nocturnal haemoglobinuria

TREATMENT

Treatment with high dose warfarin (INR >3) is
the most effective way of controlling the
syndrome, reducing the risk of a second
event much more than aspirin or low dose
warfarin.
Low dose aspirin is efficacious in reducing the
risk of recurrent miscarriage.

PROGNOSIS

Patients with a single episode of thrombus are at
high risk of recurrent episodes without treatment,
with a median time to second episode of
18 months.

QUESTION SPOTTING

Grey case

Any combination of:

Abortion
Venous/arterial thrombosis
Low platelets
Livedo reticularis

should prompt consideration of the
antiphospholipid syndrome, as should
thrombosis in the presence of a positive VDRL.
The syndrome may accompany SLE or
another autoimmune disease as part of a dual
diagnosis.

Data interpretation

The clues are:

Presence of a thrombosis or abortion
Low platelets
Prolonged APTT
Positive VDRL

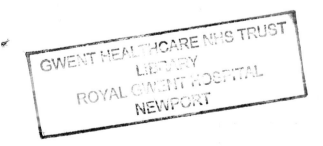

LYMPHOMA

A heterogeneous group of disorders caused by a proliferation of various cells in the lymphoid system, classified as Hodgkin's disease (HD) or non-Hodgkin's lymphoma (NHL). Further classification of HD can be seen in Table 1 and the staging of this disease, which is important for treatment, is seen in Table 2. NHL has a complicated classification and depends on the rate of cell division, the cell type involved and the behaviour of the disease. The two most frequently used classifications are the Working Formulation which has low grade, intermediate grade and high grade, while the Kiel Classification divides the condition into low grade and high grade and T cell and B cell. The details of these classifications are not important for the MRCP examination.

Table 1 Rye classification of Hodgkin's disease

Type	Frequency	Prognosis
Nodular sclerosing	64%	Good
Lymphocyte depleted	2%	Poor
Mixed cellularity	25%	Good
Lymphocyte predominance	6%	Good
Unclassified	3%	

Table 2 Ann Arbor staging system

Stage	
I	Single LN region (I) or extralymphatic organ (Ie)
II	2 or more LN regions on same side of diaphragm (II) or 1 or more LN regions with an extralymphatic organ (IIe)
III	LN regions on both sides of the diaphragm (III)
IV	2 or more extralymphatic organs (IV)
Subtype	
A	Asymptomatic
B	Type B symptoms of fever, night sweats, >10% weight loss

SYMPTOMS

Lymph node enlargement
Fever
Weight loss
Night sweats
Possible shortness of breath, lethargy due to anaemia
Recurrent infections due to lymphopenia
Bleeding due to thrombocytopenia
Alcohol induced lymph node pain is characteristic but rare
Pruritus
Fits, neurological symptoms (CNS lymphoma)

SIGNS

Fever
Lymphadenopathy
Abdominal mass
Hepatomegaly
Splenomegaly
Focal neurological signs

INVESTIGATIONS

FBC
Hb usually normal but may be ↓
WCC ↑ or ↓ (↓ is poor prognostic sign).
   Eosinophilia may occur
Platelets usually normal, but may be ↓
ESR usually raised

U + Es
Na normal
K normal
Urea and creatinine may ↑ if ureteric obstruction from lymphadenopathy

LFTs
Bilirubin ↑
AST ↑
ALP ↑ (may ↑ due to liver or bony disease)
Calcium ↑ if bony disease
Uric acid ↑
LDH ↑

Chest X-ray
Hilar enlargement

DIAGNOSIS

Lymph node biopsy
Bone marrow biopsy and trephine
CT scan of chest, abdomen and pelvis
Lumbar puncture

DIFFERENTIAL DIAGNOSIS

Causes of lymphadenopathy include
Lymphoma
Metastatic malignancy
Infective: bacterial (pyogenic, TB, brucella),
    fungal, viral (HIV, EBV, CMV) and parasitic
    (syphilis, toxoplasma)
Reactive: sarcoid, rheumatoid arthritis and other
    connective tissue diseases, eczema, psoriasis,
    drugs (phenytoin, berylliosis)
Infiltrative: lipidosis, histiocytosis

COMPLICATIONS

Complications tend to occur due to treatment

Radiotherapy
Radiation lung fibrosis
Cardiomyopathy
Hypothyroidism

Chemotherapy
Alopecia
Infertility
Neurotoxicity
Aseptic bone necrosis
Infections
Secondary malignancies
Progressive multifocal leucoencephalopathy
Tumour lysis syndrome

TREATMENT

Depends on staging of disease:

Radiotherapy
Extended field, external beam radiotherapy is
used particularly in stage Ia and IIa disease. All
lymph node groups are treated in the affected
half of the body and additional doses are given to
node groups known to be involved. Radiotherapy
may also have a place in Ib, IIb and IIIa
disease.

Chemotherapy
Used in more disseminated disease. ChlVPP
(chlorambucil, vinblastine, procarbazine and
prednisolone) the most common regimens or
ABVD (adriamycin, bleomycin, vinblastine and
dacarbazine) are in use for HD, whilst CHOP
(chlorambucil, adriamycin, vincristine and
prednisolone) is the most used in high grade
NHL. Single agents may be used in low grade
disease.

Bone marrow transplant
May play a part, but long-term outcome is still
not clear, and there is still a high mortality rate
associated with this treatment.

PROGNOSIS

80% 5 year survival in HD, though this depends
on the histology. NHL carries a worse overall
prognosis, maybe due to the variety of disease;
80% show initial response to treatment, but only
35% are still disease free at 5 years.

QUESTION SPOTTING

Grey case
Lymphoma may commonly present in this
section of the examination, since it may easily be
confused with infective or malignant causes of
lymphadenopathy. The most important
diagnostic test is a lymph node biopsy which
should give the diagnosis.

Data interpretation
Less likely to crop up in this section.

LEUKAEMIAS

Malignant haemopoietic disorder characterized by unregulated proliferation of one stem line which is usually nonfunctional. These abnormal cells replace the normal bone marrow including haemopoietic precursors and this results in the loss of other cell lines. Usually the cause is not known, but documented aetiological factors include:

Hereditary, e.g. Down's syndrome, ataxia telangiectasia, Wiskott-Aldrich syndrome
Chemicals, e.g. benzene, alkylating agents
Radiation exposure
Myelodysplasia
Aplastic anaemia
Viral infection, e.g. HTLV-1

The leukaemias are divided into acute and chronic and they are also divided according to which cell line is affected. The classification is shown in Table 1.

The typical age of incidence varies for each type of leukaemia. Although all types may occur at any age, the most typical presentation of ALL is at 2–10 years old with a smaller rise in incidence over 40 years. AML increases with age: the median age is 60. Peak incidence of CML is 40–60 years and CLL almost always occurs after 60.

Table 1 Classification of the leukaemias

Acute lymphoblastic leukaemia	Acute myeloid leukaemia*
Undifferentiated	M0 undifferentiated
Pre-B	M1 minimal differentiation
B cell	M2 differentiated
T cell	M3 promyelocytic
	M4 myelomonocytic
	M5 monocytic
	M6 erythrocytic
	M7 megakaryocytic
Chronic lymphocytic leukaemia	Chronic myeloid leukaemia
Classical B cell	Philadelphia positive
Prolymphocytic cell	Philadelphia negative
Hairy cell	

*FAB (French, American, British) classification

SYMPTOMS

Anaemia causing tiredness, lethargy and dyspnoea.
Neutropenia causing recurrent infections.
Thrombocytopenia causing spontaneous bruising, menorrhagia, gingival bleeding and nose bleeds.
Others: weight loss, abdominal pain and bloating, anorexia, night sweats, recurrent ulcers, bone pain, and gum hyperplasia (especially in M5 AML).

SIGNS

Fever
Pallor
Petechial haemorrhages, purpura and fundal haemorrhages
Hepatomegaly
Splenomegaly
Peripheral lymphadenopathy

INVESTIGATIONS

FBC
Hb $\downarrow$ (MCV normal)
WCC may be $\uparrow\uparrow$ or $\downarrow\downarrow$ (range $<1.0 \times 10^9$ to $>200 \times 10^9$). Differential often abnormal.
Platelets $\downarrow$ (often $<10 \times 10^9$/L)

U + Es
K + $\uparrow$ especially in tumour lysis syndrome
Urea and creatinine $\uparrow$ if renal impairment

LFTs
Bilirubin may be $\uparrow$
Albumin $\downarrow$
ALP $\uparrow$
ALT $\uparrow$
Total protein $\downarrow$ in CLL
Immunoglobulins often $\downarrow$ in CLL (but may be $\uparrow$ with a monoclonal band on electrophoresis)
Urate $\uparrow$ in acute leukaemias and occasionally in CML and as part of the tumour lysis syndrome
LDH $\uparrow$ in acute leukaemias
Coagulation often abnormal (M3 AML is predisposed to DIC)
Coombs' test often positive in CLL

Chest X-ray

Mediastinal mass may occur (especially in T cell ALL)

Lytic bony lesions may be seen

DIAGNOSIS

Blood film
Bone marrow examination
Cytogenetics
Cytochemistry
Immunophenotyping
Lumbar puncture to detect CNS involvement

DIFFERENTIAL DIAGNOSIS

Lymphoma and infection for lymphadenopathy
Myeloproliferative disorders, myelodysplasia, autoimmune disease and infection may all cause hepatosplenomegaly
Aplastic anaemia or bone marrow infiltration if pancytopenia

AML may be difficult to differentiate from polycythemia rubra vera and myelofibrosis.

TREATMENT

Supportive

Transfusions of blood, platelets, FFP and cryoprecipitate.
Antibiotics for infections – regimens vary from unit to unit. Multiple cultures are essential to target the causative organism and infection site.
Barrier nursing while neutropenic.
Psychological support.

Radiotherapy

May be indicated in the elderly with CLL

Chemotherapy

Allopurinol prior to starting chemotherapy to prevent acute gout and renal impairment.
Intravenous hydration to prevent renal impairment.
Cycles of chemotherapy given to induce and consolidate remission.
Maintenance therapy may then be given. CNS prophylaxis is often required especially with

ALL. Specific regimens vary and will not be discussed here.

Bone marrow transplantation

Allogeneic transplant may be curative in 50–60% but high morbidity and mortality (30%).
Autologous transplant not curative but lower morbidity and mortality.

Other

Splenectomy may be useful if haemolytic anaemia or gross splenic enlargement.

PROGNOSIS

ALL

50% long-term remission. Poorer outlook seen in early relapse, CNS disease and testicular disease, high WCC at presentation, T cell disease and <1 year or >10 years of age.

AML

40% 5 year survival in younger patients. Poorer outlook seen in early relapse, CNS disease (rare), high WCC at presentation, >20% blasts in bone marrow after first course of treatment, or >60 years of age.

CLL

Median survival of 6 years. Poorer prognosis if anaemic and/or thrombocytopenic regardless of lymphoid enlargement.

CML

Median survival of 4–5 years. Poorer prognosis if Philadelphia negative.

QUESTION SPOTTING

Grey case

Although a leukaemia may well present in the grey cases, you are unlikely to see a white count of more than 50×10^9. This leads to diagnostic difficulty, especially if there is a possibility of chronic infection, inflammation or infarction that could give a reactive leukocytosis. However do remember that ineffective leukocytosis in leukaemic patients predisposes to recurrent infections.

Data interpretation

Less likely to appear in this section.

MULTIPLE MYELOMA

Malignant proliferation of plasma cells (B lymphocytes). The monoclonal plasma cell line produces large quantities of immunoglobulin in most cases, and cytokine interactions between the malignant cells and the bone marrow lead to suppression of normal immunoglobulin production, enhanced osteoclastic activity, and suppression of normal blood cell production.

SYMPTOMS

Often insidious in onset; 20% are asymptomatic
Bone pain
Tiredness
Weight loss
SOB
Fever (uncommon)
Infection, e.g. pneumonia
Thirst, polyuria

SIGNS

Pallor
Signs of infection

INVESTIGATIONS

FBC
Hb ↓ (in 60%)
MCV normal
WCC may be ↓
Platelets may be ↓

U + Es
Urea and creatinine raised in 20%

LFTs
Albumin often ↓ (especially in advanced disease)
Total protein usually ↑
ALP normal (unless bone fracture)

ESR ↑ in 90%
CRP often normal, but may be ↑
Calcium ↑ (in 30%)
INR, APTTR usually normal
Anion gap ↓
Blood film shows rouleaux. Plasma cells in 5%

X-rays
Lytic lesions in 60% (sclerotic lesions are rare). Usually in the axial skeleton
Osteoporosis (without lytic lesions in 20%)

Bone scan normal (unless fractures)

Immunoglobulins
Monoclonal gammopathy – IgG (60%), IgA (20–25%), IgD and non-secreting types (rare)
Light chains only in 15–20%
Other Ig levels are suppressed
Urine may show Bence–Jones proteinuria
Bone marrow shows excess plasma cells, often with multiple nuclei

DIAGNOSIS

A secure diagnosis needs one major plus one minor criterion, or three minor criteria:

Major
Plasmacytoma
>30% plasma cells on bone marrow biopsy
Monoclonal Ig: >35 g/L IgG, >20 g/L IgA
>1 g/24 h of Bence-Jones protein

Minor
>10% plasma cells on bone marrow biopsy
Monoclonal Ig
Lytic lesions on skeletal survey (not bone scan)
Immune paresis: IgM <0.5 g/L, IgA <1 g/L, IgG <6 g/L

DIFFERENTIAL DIAGNOSIS

Monoclonal gammopathy of undetermined significance (MGUS)
Chronic lymphocytic leukaemia
Lymphoma
Vasculitis
Primary amyloidosis
Other metastatic malignancy

COMPLICATIONS

Bone fractures
Infections, particularly pneumococcal
Hypercalcaemia
Renal failure
Amyloidosis (AL type)
Coagulopathy
Neuropathy
Hyperviscosity syndrome (usually with IgA)
Soft tissue plasmacytoma
Spinal cord compression

PROGNOSIS

Median survival 10 months without treatment
Median survival 2–3 years with melphalan

Adverse prognostic indicators include:
Hb <8.5 g/dL
Hypercalcaemia
Renal impairment
β_2 microglobulin > 6 g/L
Very high Ig levels
Advanced lytic lesions

TREATMENT

Rehydration, steroids and bisphosphonates for
   hypercalcaemia
Analgesia and radiotherapy for bone pain
Rehydration +/– dialysis for renal impairment
Transfusion for anaemia
Melphalan with prednisolone can usually induce
   a partial remission.

High dose chemotherapy with bone marrow
   transplantation may prolong survival, but has a
   mortality of 40% and is not usually offered to
   those over 55 years of age.

QUESTION SPOTTING

Grey case

Myeloma presents as an insidious illness with
non-specific features; suspect in anyone with
tiredness, lethargy, thirst, back pain or recurrent
infections. Osteoporosis in a man should also
alert you to this diagnosis.

Data interpretation

Look out for the following:

High ESR with normal CRP
High protein gap (total protein – albumin)
High calcium plus normocytic anaemia,
   especially in the context of renal
   impairment

WALDENSTRÖM'S MACROGLOBULINAEMIA

Monoclonal plasma cell neoplasm, producing large quantities of monoclonal IgM. This leads to the hyperviscosity syndrome, as well as suppression of normal bone marrow activity. Unlike multiple myeloma, disruption of osteoclast activity is not usually a feature, and hypercalcaemia and renal impairment are uncommon.

CLINICAL FEATURES

General
Weight loss
Lethargy
Shortness of breath
Hepatomegaly
Splenomegaly
Lymphadenopathy
Mucosal bleeding

Hyperviscosity syndrome (occurs in 70%)
Visual loss or impairment
Reduced conscious level
Seizures
Ataxia, vertigo, neuropathy
Retinal vein distension ('sausage string' appearance) and haemorrhage
Cardiac failure (due to increased plasma volume)
DVT, PE

Other features
10% show evidence of lung or skin infiltration

IgM cryoglobulinaemia
Raynaud's phenomenon
Digital gangrene
Arthralgia
Haemolytic anaemia
Vascular purpura
Amyloid (10–15%)

INVESTIGATIONS

FBC
Hb ↓
MCV normal
WCC may be ↓
Lymphocytes ↑ in late disease
Platelets may be ↓
Reticulocytes may be ↑

U + Es
Usually normal

LFTs
Bilirubin ↑ if haemolysis
Total protein ↑
Otherwise normal
Calcium normal
ESR very ↑
LDH may be ↑
Immunoglobulins show ↑ IgM; monoclonal band on electrophoresis
X-rays show no osteoporosis or lytic lesions
Urine shows Bence-Jones protein in 70%
Bone marrow shows excess numbers of lymphoplasmacytoid cells

DIAGNOSIS

Presence of IgM paraprotein (monoclonal) together with neoplastic plasma cells in bone marrow. Lytic lesions of bone are almost always absent.

DIFFERENTIAL DIAGNOSIS

For IgM paraprotein
MGUS (see myeloma)
Non-Hodgkin's lymphoma
Chronic lymphocytic leukaemia
Primary amyloidosis

For hyperviscosity syndrome
Myeloma
Polycythaemia rubra vera
CML
AML

TREATMENT

Hyperviscosity syndrome requires plasmapheresis for treatment.
Chlorambucil or melphalan can be used to reduce paraprotein levels and thus improve symptoms.

PROGNOSIS

Median survival is 6 years.

QUESTION SPOTTING

Grey case

Look for:

Normocytic anaemia

High total protein

Symptoms of headache, coma or visual disturbance

Raynaud's phenomenon

Hepatosplenomegaly

Note that bone pain, hypercalcaemia and renal impairment suggest myeloma rather than Waldenström's disease.

Data interpretation

Raised total protein, normocytic anaemia with normal calcium and renal function are the clues. A very high ESR (>150) also suggests Waldenström's.

MISCELLANEOUS

10

The toxic effects of tricyclic antidepressants are myriad, due to the multiple pharmacological actions of these drugs. These actions include catecholamine uptake inhibition, anticholinergic effects, and fast sodium channel blockade. Cardiac and CNS toxicity are responsible for fatalities, which currently run at an average of one per day in the UK.

CLINICAL FEATURES

Cardiovascular
Tachycardia
Hypotension
SVT, VT, VF
Heart block
Pulmonary oedema

Neurological
Lethargy
Coma
Hyperreflexia
Seizures
Hallucinations
Ataxia
Loss of brainstem reflexes
Respiratory depression

Autonomic
Dry mouth
Urinary retention
Pyrexia or hypothermia
Dilated pupils
Constipation

Unusual features
Rhabdomyolysis (esp. if prolonged seizures)
Skin blisters
DIC
Peripheral neuropathy

INVESTIGATIONS

FBC
Usually normal

U + Es
Sodium usually normal
Potassium may be $\downarrow$
Urea and creatinine normal

LFTs
ALT may be $\uparrow$
Otherwise normal
Clotting usually normal

CK may be $\uparrow$ (skeletal and cardiac)
ABGs show metabolic or mixed acidosis
ECG shows sinus tachycardia, ST/T wave changes, QT prolongation, PR prolongation, QRS prolongation. QRS >100 ms carries a much higher chance of dangerous arrhythmias. RBBB, AV block, SVT, VT, torsade or VF may develop

TREATMENT

Protect airway if at risk
100% O_2
Cardiac monitoring for at least 6 h
Gastric lavage if severe overdose within 1–2 h
50–100 g charcoal, repeated at 2–4 h if severe overdose
Treat convulsions with diazepam
Sodium bicarbonate if acidosis, QRS widening, low BP or arrhythmias, other signs of severe toxicity. Aim for arterial pH of 7.45–7.55
Aim for K^+ at upper end of normal
IV colloid/crystalloid for hypotension; consider glucagon in refractory cases

Arrhythmias
Sodium bicarbonate and oxygen.
DC shock if refractory.
Avoid antiarrhythmics if possible, but consider phenytoin, lignocaine, atenolol or esmolol.
If cardiac arrest occurs, resuscitation attempts should continue for longer than usual; good recovery has been observed after 2–5 h CPR in tricyclic overdoses.
Class Ia and Ic antiarrhythmics are contraindicated, as are physostigmine and flumazenil (in mixed overdose). Dialysis and charcoal haemoperfusion are ineffective at removing tricyclic antidepressants.

PROGNOSIS

2–3% mortality rate. Serious complications usually occur within 6 h of ingestion (peak plasma levels are usually around 4 h). Onset of seizures or arrhythmias is extremely rare after 24 h.

QUESTION SPOTTING

Grey case

This topic could occur in a grey case; the fact that an overdose has been taken is usually obvious. The key features are usually:
Dilated pupils
Reduced level of consciousness
Tachycardia

The neurological sequelae of fits or arrhythmias can make the diagnosis more difficult, with head injury or intracranial haemorrhage entering the differential.

Data interpretation

The clues here are an acidosis with a normal osmolality (cf. methanol or ethylene glycol overdose), normal glucose and sodium and perhaps a low potassium. The ECG changes may be shown.

LEAD POISONING

Acute lead poisoning is a rare event. However, chronic toxicity is more common, and is particularly seen in certain situations:

Industrial – metal workers, smelting workers.
Domestic – drinking water from lead pipes, children ingesting lead based paints.

SYMPTOMS

Anorexia
Nausea and vomiting
Muscle weakness
Constipation
Abdominal colic, which may mimic an acute abdomen
Behaviour change
Seizures
Memory loss

SIGNS

Blue line around gums – due to deposition of sulphide.
Peripheral neuropathy which is almost exclusively motor, and particularly affects extensors, leading to wrist and foot drop.

INVESTIGATIONS

FBC
Hb normal or ↓ – may be normochromic, normocytic, sideroblastic or even haemolytic
WCC normal
Platelets normal

U + Es
Urea and creatinine ↑ if nephritis

LFTs
Normal
Blood film may show basophilic stippling
Erythrocyte protoporphyrin ↑, and ↓ ALA dehydratase activity seen

Urine
Glycosuria
Proteinuria – aminoaciduria

Long bone X-rays
Dense metaphyseal bands, especially wrists and knees in children

DIAGNOSIS

Urine
↑ ALA and ↑ coproporphyrin
Serum lead ↑
Urine lead excretion ↑

ASSOCIATIONS

Gout

DIFFERENTIAL DIAGNOSIS

May be confused with acute intermittent porphyria

COMPLICATIONS

Interstitial nephritis – tubular dysfunction may lead to glycosuria, phosphaturia, aminoaciduria due to reduced absorption. This is reversible if caught early, but irreversible once fibrosis has occurred.

TREATMENT

Remove cause
Calcium EDTA, D-penicillamine or dimercaprol to chelate the lead
Monitor U + Es

QUESTION SPOTTING

Grey case
Think of this in the non-surgical causes of abdominal pain. Now very rare. Also consider it if glycosuria in a young patient, especially if anaemic, and occupational exposure particularly in an unregulated industry.

Data interpretation
Unlikely to appear in this section.

DIGOXIN TOXICITY

Digoxin is thought to inhibit the action of the Na^+/K^+ ATPase of the sarcolemmal membrane. This causes sodium influx and displacement of bound intra-cellular calcium giving a positive inotropic effect. Digoxin also causes an increased refractory period and slows conduction at the AV node. Other effects include mild peripheral vasoconstriction, a vagotonic effect, and increased cardiac automaticity.

Because of its diversity of actions and its complicated pharmacokinetics, digoxin toxicity is a clinical diagnosis, but may often be confirmed by toxic concentrations in the blood.

Factors that increase cardiac sensitivity to digoxin

$\downarrow$ K (but $\uparrow$ K may cause heart block)
$\downarrow$ Mg
$\uparrow$ Ca
Acidosis
Hypothyroidism
Cardiac amyloid
Chronic lung disease
Ischaemic cardiomyopathy
Renal impairment – causes increased plasma concentration

Drugs which interact with digoxin

Increase
Quinidine – $\downarrow$ renal clearance
Captopril – $\downarrow$ renal clearance
Amiodarone – $\downarrow$ renal clearance
Propafenone – $\downarrow$ renal clearance
Verapamil – displaced protein binding
Nifedipine – displaced protein binding
Nitrendipine – displaced protein binding
Erythromycin – $\downarrow$ bacteria in gut which convert digoxin to inactive dihydrodigoxin
Tetracycline – $\downarrow$ bacteria in gut which convert digoxin to inactive dihydrodigoxin

Decrease
Cholestyramine – binds digoxin in resin
Phenytoin – $\uparrow$ hepatic metabolism
Rifampicin – $\uparrow$ hepatic metabolism
Sulphasalazine – delayed absorption
Neomycin – delayed absorption

CLINICAL FEATURES

Non-cardiac
Fatigue
Anorexia
Nausea and vomiting
Xanthopsia
Headaches
Abdominal pain and diarrhoea
Paraesthesia
Fits
Mental confusion
Hallucinations

Cardiac
Bradycardia – either in sinus rhythm or in AF
2nd or 3rd degree AV block due to increased parasympathetic and reduced sympathetic tone
Junctional bradycardias
Paroxysmal atrial tachycardia with variable block
Ventricular ectopics, bigemini, and paroxysmal ventricular tachycardia
Ventricular fibrillation

INVESTIGATIONS

FBC
Normal

U + Es
Na normal
K normal or $\uparrow$. Digoxin toxicity worse if K $\downarrow$
Urea and creatinine normal or may be increased
Magnesium may be $\downarrow$
Ca may be $\uparrow$

DIAGNOSIS

The diagnosis is clinical
Digoxin concentrations – provide a rough guide
ECG may show the features mentioned under cardiac features. See example ECG of digoxin toxicity (Fig. 16)

TREATMENT

ECG monitoring.
Drug withdrawal.
Treatment of electrolyte disturbances. Potassium administration may be useful for the treatment

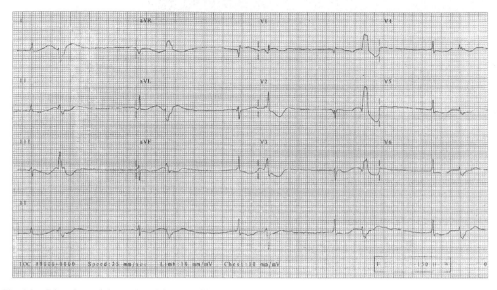

Fig. 16.   Digoxin toxicity. This ECG shows bigemini with marked bradycardia. The QRS complexes are variable in morphology and there is widespread ST segment depression with T wave abnormality.

of ventricular arrhythmias even if serum potassium levels are normal, but this requires extreme care.

Atropine is useful for sinus bradycardias, AV block, and sinoatrial arrest, although temporary pacing may be required.

Digoxin-specific antibody fragments are used for serious arrhythmias such as VT. They give rapid and selective digoxin reversal. Improvement occurs within about 30 min, and toxicity is resolved within 3–4 h. They can be used more than once in the same patient, but side effects should be watched for. VT may also be treated with lignocaine, phenytoin, amiodarone or beta blockers. Note that beta blockers may lead to heart block, and so very short acting intravenous forms such as esmolol should be used.

DC cardioversion should be avoided as it may precipitate asystole.

Haemodialysis and haemoperfusion are ineffective in clearing digoxin.

If toxicity is the result of overdose, then gastric lavage and activated charcoal are both useful treatments. Cholestyramine is also effective at binding digoxin and reducing serum concentrations.

QUESTION SPOTTING

Grey case

Suspect digoxin toxicity if unexplained nausea and vomiting, or arrhythmias, especially 2nd or 3rd degree heart block. Dimorphic VT or atrial tachycardia should also raise the suspicion of digoxin toxicity, especially in the elderly after recent introduction of a new drug – see above list.

Data interpretation

Unlikely to appear in this section.

Although pregnancy is not a disease, it may crop up in the data interpretation section, as it causes physiological changes such as:

Plasma volume expands by 30 to 40%
Cardiac output increases as result of increased rate and stroke volume
GFR increases
A number of acute phase proteins increase, including fibrinogen, transferrin and thyroid binding globulin; albumin production decreases

INVESTIGATIONS

FBC
Hb ↓ by 1 g/dL
WCC is usually normal
Platelets drop to between 90 and 150 in 5%
MCV ↑ 4 fl on average

U + Es
Urea and creatinine both fall

LFTs
ALP rises especially in 3rd trimester
ALT, AST, Igs and GGT are usually normal
Albumin is reduced by 20%

ESR rises
Folate usually falls
Fe falls to two-thirds normal
TIBC doubles

Ferritin falls to between 15 and 20
Clotting studies are usually normal
Cholesterol and triglycerides are elevated

Hormones
Total T_4 is raised, but free T_4 is normal, as is TSH
ACTH, cortisol, prolactin and renin are all elevated
GH, FSH and LH are all reduced

Urine
Glycosuria is sometimes present
Asymptomatic bacteriuria occurs in 2% to 7%
ECG may show criteria of LVH, T wave inversion in leads V2 and V3

Lung tidal volume is increased, but residual volume is reduced.

QUESTION SPOTTING

Grey case
Unlikely to appear in this section.

Data Interpretation
Pregnancy can crop up in the data interpretation section; the clue is a young woman with a selection of odd blood results that do not appear to fit any particular disease.

Note that the diagnosis of anaemia is complex in pregnancy, as most of the normal ranges for haematinics are altered.

ETHYLENE GLYCOL POISONING

Ethylene glycol poisoning usually arises from ingestion of antifreeze which contains >90% ethylene glycol, often taken with ethanol. It is colourless, odourless and slightly sweet tasting. It does not directly cause toxicity, but it is metabolized to glycolic acid by alcohol dehydrogenase. Further metabolism eventually to give calcium oxalate is slow, and so glycolic acid accumulates. Glycolate causes generalized oedema, severe acidosis, interstitial nephritis with oxalate crystal deposition and multi-organ failure.

Stages

Early (30 mins – 12 h)
Alcohol like effects and effects of hypocalcaemia.

Intermediate (12–48 h)
Severe acidosis, cardiorespiratory failure with pulmonary oedema, ARDS and gastric aspiration.

Late (48 + h)
Renal failure secondary to direct toxicity and calcium oxalate deposition.

SYMPTOMS

Disinhibition
Ataxia
Incoordination
Reduced conscious level
Fits

SIGNS

Tachycardia
Hypertension
Tachypnoea (Kussmaul respiration)
Hypotonia
Hyporeflexia
Myoclonic jerks
Fits
Absent pupillary reflexes
Papilloedema
Meningism
Coma
Oliguria/anuria

INVESTIGATIONS

FBC
Hb normal
WCC ↑
Platelets normal

U + Es
Na ↑
K normal or ↑
Urea ↑
Creatinine ↑

LFTs
Usually normal

Calcium ↓
Glucose normal or mildly ↑
Chloride normal
Anion gap ↑
Ethylene glycol levels ↑
Osmolar gap ↑ (calculated osmolality minus measured osmolality) – not explained by alcohol

ABGs
pH ↓↓
CO_2 ↓
O_2 ↓
HCO_3 ↓
BE ↓
Urine ketones negative (weak ketonuria may be seen in chronic alcoholics). Oxalate crystalluria from 8 h.
Chest X-ray shows oedema or ARDS.

DIAGNOSIS

Clinical features
Increased anion gap
Raised ethylene glycol levels with calcium oxalate crystalluria

DIFFERENTIAL DIAGNOSIS

Diabetic ketoacidosis
Methanol poisoning
Ethanol poisoning
Lactic acidosis
Ecstasy overdose
Amitriptyline overdose

COMPLICATIONS

Multiple organ failure
Hypocalcaemia secondary to sequestration by
    oxalate

TREATMENT

Airway management and resuscitation with
    fluids and inotropes if required
Gastric lavage and activated charcoal
Ethanol – competitively inhibits ethylene glycol
    metabolism with alcohol dehydrogenase
    (80 × the affinity). Levels should be titrated to
    100 mg/dL.
Sodium bicarbonate may be required for
    profound acidosis. Very large quantities may
    be required to raise pH. Note that this may
    increase calcium oxalate crystal deposition
    and renal damage.
Haemodialysis is the best method of directly
    removing ethylene glycol and its products, but
    peritoneal dialysis is effective, if slower.

PROGNOSIS

Renal failure is usually reversible with renal
    support, but may take 6–8 weeks to
    recover.
Very high mortality rates if late
    presentation/diagnosis or high doses
    taken.

QUESTION SPOTTING

Grey case
The typical patient will be young and male and
will often have a history of alcohol abuse or
previous psychiatric history. Watch out for severe
unexplained acidosis.

Data interpretation
One of the causes of high anion gap acidosis,
this may present in the data section. You
must work out the anion gap if given chloride
levels.

ECSTASY INGESTION

Ecstasy is the popular name for an amphetamine derivative (3,4-methylenedioxymethamphetamine or MDMA) which is increasing in popularity in the UK. It is taken for its stimulant and hallucinogenic properties which give feelings of euphoria, closeness and distorted sensory perceptions. Unfortunately ecstasy has been associated with some idiosyncratic and serious adverse reactions, even at doses previously tolerated, particularly when associated with dehydration and pyrexia from dancing.

SYMPTOMS

Excitement
Restlessness
Shortness of breath

SIGNS

Hypertension
Hyperventilation
Tachycardia
Hyperreflexia
Dilated pupils
Hyperpyrexia

INVESTIGATIONS

FBC
Hb normal
WCC may be normal or ↑
Platelets ↓ if DIC

U + Es
Na may be ↓↓
K ↑ if rhabdomyolysis and/or renal failure
Urea may be ↑
Creatinine may be ↑

LFTs
ALT may be ↑
ALP may be ↑
Bilirubin may be ↑
Albumin usually normal
Ca may be ↓
Clotting abnormal if DIC

ABGs
pH may be ↓
CK ↑↑ if rhabdomyolysis

Urine
Blood ++ to dipstix but no red cells on microscopy if myoglobinuria from rhabdomyolysis

DIAGNOSIS

MDMA levels may be taken to confirm clinical diagnosis

COMPLICATIONS

Cardiac
Hypotension
Ventricular arrhythmias
Myocardial infarction
Aortic dissection
Shock

Respiratory
Adult respiratory distress syndrome

Renal
Acute renal failure

Hepatic
Acute hepatic necrosis

Neurological
Paranoid psychosis
Intracranial haemorrhage

Metabolic
Malignant hyperpyrexia
Hyponatraemia

Musculoskeletal
Rhabdomyolysis

Haematological
Disseminated intravascular coagulation

TREATMENT

Supportive – fluids and ECG monitoring.
Diazepam if agitated or fitting.
Treat complications as they arise.

QUESTION SPOTTING

Grey case

Ecstasy ingestion should be suspected in any young patient who presents with signs of adrenergic stimulation, especially if multiple organ failure. The typical patient will be in their teens or early 20s with dilated pupils, tachycardia, hyperventilation and restlessness. Fitting, cardiac arrhythmias, rhabdomyolysis and DIC seem to be typical severe complications.

Data interpretation

Not suitable for this section.

PRE-ECLAMPSIA

This is a pregnancy specific multi-system disorder characterized by hypertension, proteinuria, thrombocytopenia, renal dysfunction and abnormal liver function. The actual cause remains unknown, but there appears to be diffuse endothelial dysfunction affecting all organs and particularly the placenta which becomes ischaemic. Imbalance occurs between prostacyclin ($\downarrow$) and thromboxane A2 ($\uparrow$), and there is defective production of nitric oxide. There is a wide variation in clinical presentation, but the classic triad is hypertension, proteinuria and oedema.

The disease usually occurs late in the first pregnancy, and risk factors include:

Increasing age
Family history
Pre-pregnancy hypertension
Pre-pregnancy renal disease
Antiphospholipid syndrome
Diabetes mellitus
Twin gestation

SYMPTOMS

May be asymptomatic
Headache
Visual disturbance, e.g. flashing lights
Ankle oedema
Abdominal pains
Nausea and vomiting

SIGNS

Hypertension
Tachycardia
Oedema
Proteinuria
Confusion
Hyperreflexia
Papilloedema (late)

INVESTIGATIONS

FBC
Hb $\uparrow$
WCC normal
Platelets $\downarrow$
Haematocrit $\uparrow$

U + Es
Na normal
K normal
Urea $\uparrow$
Creatinine $\uparrow$

LFTs
AST $\uparrow$
ALT $\uparrow$
ALP $\uparrow$ (no more than is normal in pregnancy)
Bilirubin $\uparrow$
Albumin $\downarrow$ or $\downarrow\downarrow$

Clotting
PT may be $\uparrow$
APTT may be $\uparrow$
Uric acid $\uparrow$ (rises earlier than urea and creatinine)
Lactic acid dehydrogenase $\uparrow$

Blood film
Microangiopathic haemolytic anaemia

DIAGNOSIS

Hypertension (systolic >140 mmHg and >30 mmHg over baseline and diastolic >90 mmHg and >15 mmHg over baseline)
Urinary protein >0.3 g/24 h

DIFFERENTIAL DIAGNOSIS

Essential hypertension
Pregnancy induced hypertension (no proteinuria or other features of pre-eclampsia)
HELLP syndrome (haemolysis, elevated liver enzymes, low platelets)

COMPLICATIONS

Eclampsia – seizures (presenting symptom in 30%)
Cardiac failure with pulmonary oedema
Renal failure
Hepatic failure
Hepatic rupture
Cerebral haemorrhage
Placental abruption
ARDS
DIC
Fetal death

Maternal death (stroke is commonest cause)

TREATMENT

Prophylaxis of at risk patients with low dose aspirin 75 mg/day preferably for 12 weeks prior to conception.

Control of blood pressure (most aim to keep systolic pressure <140 mmHg and diastolic <90 mmHg). Therapies used include methyldopa, nifedipine, labetalol and hydralazine. Avoid diuretics.

Severe hypertension should be treated with arterial pressure monitoring, intravenous hydralazine or labetalol.

Avoid general anaesthesia. Avoid ergotamine which increases blood pressure. Avoid diuretics for oliguria.

Delivery of foetus.

Indications for delivery
Uncontrolled blood pressure
Eclampsia
Foetal distress
Intrauterine growth retardation
Worsening maternal renal/hepatic/coagulation function

Maternal symptoms

Management of eclampsia is with magnesium sulphate intravenously by loading dose and infusion.

Postpartum monitoring as hypertension, eclampsia and oliguria may all worsen following delivery.

PROGNOSIS

Second most common cause of death in pregnancy.

10% risk of developing pre-eclampsia in the subsequent pregnancies with the same father.

QUESTION SPOTTING

Grey case
Any suggestion of hypertension or oedema in a pregnant woman should alert you to the possibility of this diagnosis. Make sure that you know the treatment of this medical emergency.

Data interpretation
Routine blood tests may suggest the diagnosis in a pregnant woman. ↑ Hb, ↓ platelets, ↑ uric acid, ↑ urea and ↑ creatinine and abnormal clotting are all highly suggestive of pre-eclampsia.

CARBON MONOXIDE POISONING

Carbon monoxide exerts its toxic effect principally by binding to haemoglobin with an avidity some 240 times that of oxygen, leading to tissue hypoxia. Secondary effects include inhibition of cytochrome oxidase activity and, possibly, peroxidation of brain lipids, which may underlie the chronic neurological sequelae of poisoning.

SYMPTOMS

Chronic or low grade poisoning
Headache
Dizziness
Fatigue
'Flu-like' symptoms

More severe poisoning
Shortness of breath
Seizures
Coma

SIGNS

Cyanosis
Reduced conscious level
Increased tone, hyperreflexia
Extensor plantars
Papilloedema
Hyperpyrexia
Crepitations in chest

NB. Cherry red skin is very unusual

Chronic neuropsychiatric sequelae (may be delayed in onset)
Cognitive impairment
Memory problems
Cortical blindness
Peripheral neuropathy
Mutism
Parkinsonism, choreoathetosis
Personality changes
Incontinence

INVESTIGATIONS

FBC
Normal

U + Es
Normal

LFTs
Normal

ABGs
pH $\downarrow$
pCO_2 $\downarrow$
pO_2 normal, but Hb saturation on ABGs
   is $\downarrow$
Pulse oximetry displays normal O_2
   saturation
ECG may show ST depression. Prolonged PR,
   QT intervals
Chest X-ray may show pulmonary oedema

DIAGNOSIS

HbCO: normal = up to 8% in smokers. Peak
   concentrations correlate with severity of
   poisoning

DIFFERENTIAL DIAGNOSIS

Drug overdose
Post ictal state
Other causes of impaired consciousness
Symptoms of chronic CO poisoning may mimic
   influenza

COMPLICATIONS

Acute renal failure
Myocardial ischaemia, arrhythmias,
   infarction
Rhabdomyolysis
TTP

TREATMENT

100% O_2
Diazepam for seizures
Mannitol and dexamethasone for cerebral
   oedema
Dantrolene for hyperpyrexia
Avoid bicarbonate as it may further impair
   oxygen release

Consider hyperbaric oxygen therapy if
Unconscious at any stage
Neurological features present
HbCO concentration >20%
Pregnant

PROGNOSIS

1500 deaths per year in UK
80% of those developing late neurological
   sequelae improve by one year after event

QUESTION SPOTTING

Grey case

You probably will not be told that the patient was found in a car with a hosepipe leading inside. Consider the diagnosis in:

Any unconscious patient
Acidosis of unknown cause
Anyone with a discrepancy between the pO_2 and Hb sats on the blood gases (not from a pulse oximeter)

Data interpretation

May also occur in this section, especially with a limited history. Do not forget the insidious presentation of chronic CO poisoning.

PHENYTOIN TOXICITY

Phenytoin toxicity occurs either acutely due to overdose, or chronically, in patients taking phenytoin regularly. Phenytoin has non-linear pharmacokinetics, highly variable oral absorption, and a variable half life that increases with plasma concentration, so toxic levels may result from minor changes in dose or in patient condition. Factors that may precipitate toxicity include hypoalbuminaemia, renal failure, hepatic dysfunction and concomitant administration of other drugs.

SYMPTOMS

Acute toxicity
Nausea and vomiting
Constipation
Slurred speech
Diplopia
Drowsiness
Confusion
Incoordination
Mood and behaviour change
Seizures (rare)
Hemi-dysaesthesia

Chronic toxicity
Gingival hyperplasia
Acne
Hirsutism

SIGNS

Acute toxicity
Bradycardia
Nystagmus
Dysarthria
Ataxia
Coarse resting tremor
Hyperreflexia with clonus
Choreoathetosis
Dyskinesia (rare)
Hemiparesis (rare)
Coma (rare)

Chronic toxicity
Lymphadenopathy

INVESTIGATIONS

FBC
Usually normal
MCV may ↑ in chronic use

U + Es
Na normal or ↓
K normal
Urea and creatinine normal

LFTs
Usually normal (rarely all may be elevated if hepatic failure)
ALP may ↑ with long-term use

Glucose ↑

ECG
Bradycardia
AV block
Idioventricular rhythm

Chest X-ray
Normal but may show signs of cardiac failure

DIAGNOSIS

Phenytoin levels ↑ (toxicity rare below 20 μg/mL)

DIFFERENTIAL DIAGNOSIS

Viral labyrinthitis
Posterior fossa tumour
Guillain-Barré syndrome
Botulism
Psychological illness

COMPLICATIONS

Cardiac failure from myocardial depression.
Cardiac arrest with VF or asystole.
Hepatic failure.
Death is rare and almost always from cardiac arrhythmias secondary to intravenous phenytoin administration.

TREATMENT

Supportive
ECG monitoring
Fluids for hypotension

Atropine for bradycardia/AV block. Cardiac pacing is occasionally required.
Haemodialysis/peritoneal dialysis are of no benefit.

PROGNOSIS

Very good once the phenytoin levels are reduced. Long-term cerebellar effects may be seen with chronic toxicity but are rare in acute overdose. Death is rare with level <70–100 mg/L.

QUESTION SPOTTING

Grey case

The patient may be either sex and any age, but the typical features of ataxia, nystagmus and drowsiness and the features of chronic use should lead to the correct diagnosis. Watch out for recent changes in medications with epileptic patients.

Data interpretation

Unlikely to appear in this section.

LITHIUM TOXICITY

Lithium is a cation handled by the body like sodium and usually administered as lithium carbonate. Toxicity may occur easily, as the therapeutic window is narrow. Excretion is completely dependent on renal function. 95% of lithium is freely filtered in the glomerulus, followed by tubular reabsorption in competition with sodium. Thus during sodium depletion, lithium is preferentially reabsorbed, and in sodium excess, more lithium is lost. Therefore in situations of salt and water depletion, there is reduced lithium excretion which leads to more salt and water loss, and this sets up a vicious circle.

This cycle may be precipitated by several drugs, but especially thiazide diuretics, non-steroidal anti-inflammatory drugs, steroids and angiotensin converting enzyme inhibitors (ACE-I). Toxicity may also occur with other causes of salt loss, e.g. diarrhoea or excess sweating due to fever, thyroid dysfunction.

CLINICAL FEATURES SEEN AT THERAPEUTIC LEVELS

Symptoms
Fine tremor
Nausea
Weight gain
Skin rash
Diarrhoea
Thirst
Polyuria

Signs
Tremor
Skin rash

CLINICAL FEATURES SEEN DURING MILD TOXICITY

Symptoms
Coarse tremor
Anorexia
Tinnitus
Drowsiness

Signs
Dysarthria

Nystagmus
Hypotension

CLINICAL FEATURES SEEN DURING SEVERE TOXICITY

Severe gastrointestinal symptoms
Seizures
Hyperreflexia and hyper-extension
Cardiac arrhythmias
Renal failure
Circulatory collapse
Coma

INVESTIGATIONS

FBC
Hb normal
WCC ↑
Platelets normal

U + Es
Na ↓
K normal, ↑ or ↓
Urea ↑
Creatinine ↑
Glucose ↑
Thyroid function: ↑ TSH, ↓ T_4

ECG
T wave flattening or inversion
ST depression
Rarely conduction defects

DIAGNOSIS

Lithium levels (levels >2.0 mmol/L are likely to be associated with toxicity)

DIFFERENTIAL DIAGNOSIS

Phenytoin overdose
Alcohol abuse
Diabetic ketoacidosis
Gastroenteritis
Other causes of diabetes insipidus
Psychogenic polydipsia

COMPLICATIONS

Nephrogenic diabetes insipidus
Hypothyroidism

Hyperglycaemia
Hyperparathyroidism

TREATMENT

Stop contributory drugs
Replace salt and water
Gastric lavage only if acute overdose
Haemodialysis is treatment of choice in severe
    intoxication with levels >3.5 mmol/L

PROGNOSIS

Mortality rates of 25% in acute overdose and 9%
in chronic toxicity. Irreversible renal impairment
may occur.

QUESTION SPOTTING

Grey case

Another cause of confusion and collapse. The
patient will have a history of depression and
some precipitating event or be on
diuretics/ACE-I.

Data interpretation

May be asked to interpret plasma and urinary
abnormalities with diabetes insipidus as a result
of lithium therapy.

ABBREVIATIONS

11

5 HIAA	5-hydroxyindoleacetic acid	CPR	Cardiopulmonary resuscitation
5 HT	5-hydroxytryptamine (serotonin)	Cr	Chromium
A&E	Accident and emergency	CREST	Calcinosis, Raynaud's,
ABGs	Arterial blood gases		oesophageal dysmotility,
ACE	Angiotensin converting		sclerodactyly and telangiectasia
	enzyme	CRF	Chronic renal failure,
AChR	Acetylcholine receptor		Corticotrophin releasing factor
ACTH	Adrenocorticotrophic hormone	CRP	C-reactive protein
ADH	Antidiuretic hormone	CSF	Cerebrospinal fluid
AF	Atrial fibrillation	CT	Computed tomography
AIDS	Acquired immune deficiency	CVA	Cerebrovascular accident
	syndrome	CXR	Chest X-ray
ALA	Aminolaevulinic acid	DI	Diabetes insipidus
ALP	Alkaline phosphatase	DIC	Disseminated intravascular
ALT	Alanine transaminase		coagulation
AML	Acute myeloid leukaemia	DKA	Diabetic ketoacidosis
ANA	Anti-nuclear antibody	DNA	Deoxyribonucleic acid
ANCA	Anti-neutrophil cytoplasmic	dsDNA	double stranded DNA
	antibody	DVT	Deep vein thrombosis
APS	Autoimmune polyglandular	EBV	Epstein-Barr virus
	syndrome	ECG	Electrocardiogram
APTT	Activated partial thromboplastin	EDTA	Ethyldiaminetetracetic acid
	time	EEG	Electroencephalogram
APUD	Amine precursor uptake and	EMG	Electromyography
	decarboxylation	ESR	Erythrocyte sedimentation rate
ARDS	Adult respiratory distress	FBC	Full blood count
	syndrome	Fe	Iron
ARF	Acute renal failure	FEV_1	Forced expiratory volume in one
ASD	Atrial septal defect		second
ASOT	Anti-streptolysin O titre	FFP	Fresh frozen plasma
AST	Aspartate transaminase	FMF	Familial Mediterranean fever
ATP	Adenosine triphosphate	FSH	Follicle stimulating hormone
ATTR	Altered transthyretin receptor	FVC	Forced vital capacity
AV	Atrioventricular, Aortic valve	GBM	Glomerular basement membrane
AXR	Abdominal X ray	GCS	Glasgow Coma Score
BAL	Bronchoalveolar lavage	GFR	Glomerular filtration rate
BE	Base excess	GGT	Gamma glutamyl transferase
BHL	Bilateral hilar lymphadenopathy	GH	Growth hormone
BP	Blood pressure	GHRH	Growth hormone releasing
cAMP	cyclic Adenosine monophosphate		hormone
CCF	Congestive cardiac failure	GI	Gastrointestinal
CK	Creatine kinase	GnRH	Gonadotrophin releasing
Cl	Chloride		hormone
CLL	Chronic lymphocytic leukaemia	GU	Genitourinary
CML	Chronic myeloid leukaemia	Hb	Haemoglobin
CMV	Cytomegalovirus	HbCO	Carboxyhaemoglobin
CNS	Central nervous system	HBsAg	Hepatitis B surface antigen
CO	Carbon monoxide	HCG	Human chorionic gonadotrophin
COPD	Chronic obstructive pulmonary	HCO_3	Bicarbonate
	disease	Hct	Haematocrit

HELLP	Haemolysis, elevated liver functions, low platelets	PBC	Primary biliary cirrhosis
		PCP	*Pneumocystis carinii* pneumonia
HIV	Human immunodeficiency virus	PCR	Polymerase chain reaction
HSV	Herpes simplex virus	PDA	Patent ductus arteriosus
HUS	Haemolytic uraemic syndrome	PE	Pulmonary embolism
IDDM	Insulin dependent diabetes mellitus	PET	Positron emission tomography
		PFTs	Pulmonary function tests
IGF 1	Insulin like growth factor	Plts	Platelets
Igs	Immunoglobulins	PNH	Paroxysmal nocturnal haemoglobinuria
IL	Interleukin		
IM	Intramuscular	PO_4	Phosphate
INR	International normalized ratio	PR	Per rectum
ITP	Idiopathic thrombocytopenic purpura	PSA	Prostate specific antigen
		PSM	Pansystolic murmur
IV	Intravenous	PTH	Parathyroid hormone
IVC	Inferior vena cava	PTHrP	PTH related peptide
IVU	Intravenous urography	PUO	Pyrexia of unknown origin
JVP	Jugular venous pressure	RA	Right atrium, Rheumatoid arthritis
K	Potassium	RBBB	Right bundle branch block
Kco	TLco corrected for lung volume	RBC	Red blood cell
kD	kilodalton	RIF	Right iliac fossa
LA	Left atrium	RNA	Ribonucleic acid
LBBB	Left bundle branch block	RNP	Ribonucleoprotein
LDH	Lactate dehydrogenase	RT	Reverse transcriptase
LFTs	Liver function tests	RTA	Renal tubular acidosis
LH	Luteinizing hormone	RUQ	Right upper quadrant
LV	Left ventricle	RV	Right ventricle
LVH	Left ventricular hypertrophy	RVH	Right ventricular hypertrophy
MAI	*Mycobacterium avium-intracellulare*	SBE	Subacute bacterial endocarditis
		SCC	Squamous cell carcinoma
MCH	Mean cell haemoglobin	SIADH	Syndrome of inappropriate antidiuretic hormone secretion
MCTD	Mixed connective tissue disease		
MCV	Mean cell volume	SLE	Systemic lupus erythematosus
MEN	Multiple endocrine neoplasia	SOB	Short of breath
Mg	Magnesium	STD	Sexually transmitted disease
MGUS	Monoclonal gammopathy of undetermined significance	SVC	Superior vena cava
		SVT	Supra-ventricular tachycardia
MI	Myocardial infarction	SXR	Skull X-ray
MIBG	Metaiodobenzylguanidine	T_3	Triiodothyronine
MRI	Magnetic resonance imaging	T_4	Thyroxine
MS	Multiple sclerosis	TB	Tuberculosis
MSU	Mid stream urine	TFTs	Thyroid function tests
Na	Sodium	TIA	Transient ischaemic attack
NSAID	Non-steroidal anti-inflammatory drug	TIBC	Total iron binding capacity
		TLco	Carbon monoxide transfer factor
OCP	Oral contraceptive pill	TNF	Tumour necrosis factor
PA	Pulmonary artery	TOE	Transoesophageal echocardiography
PABA	Para-aminobenzoic acid		
PAN	Polyarteritis nodosa	TPN	Total parenteral nutrition
PAS	Periodic acid-Schiff	TR	Tricuspid regurgitation

TSH	Thyroid stimulating hormone	VIP	Vasoactive intestinal polypeptide
TTP	Thrombotic thrombocytopenic purpura	VSD	Ventricular septal defect
		VT	Ventricular tachycardia
U + Es	Urea and electrolytes	VZV	Varicella zoster virus
UC	Ulcerative colitis	WCC	White cell count
URTI	Upper respiratory tract infection	WPW	Wolff-Parkinson-White syndrome
UTI	Urinary tract infection		
VDRL	Venereal diseases research laboratory	Zn	Zinc
		ZN	Ziehl-Nielsen (stain)
VF	Ventricular fibrillation		

QUESTIONS

12

QUESTION 1

A 30 year old woman presents with a 3 week history of a sore left eye. On direct questioning she admits to loose stools, cramping abdominal pains and mild dysuria. She is usually well, and her only medication is mouth gel for recurrent mouth ulcers. She drinks occasional alcohol, smokes 10 cigarettes per day and works as an air hostess on the route to Turkey, her native land.

On examination, she is apyrexial. She has a faint papular rash over her trunk, two aphthous ulcers and three small genital ulcers. Her left eye is red and inflamed. Pulse 80 bpm irregular, BP 120/70 mmHg. Heart sounds are normal, ankles are not swollen. Chest and abdominal exam are normal. Rectal examination reveals loose stool but no blood. Examination of her joints is unremarkable.

Investigations:
Hb 10.3 g/dL
WCC 8.1×10^9/L
Platelets 251×10^9/L
ESR 71 mm/h
CRP 30 mg/L
Rheumatoid factor negative

Questions
1) What is the most likely diagnosis?
2) Give three other possible diagnoses.
3) What test would you perform next?

QUESTION 2

These are the pressure and saturation data from the cardiac catheterization of a 16 year old boy.

Site	Pressure mmHg	Saturation %
SVC	5	65
RA	6	74
RV	25/0–5	78
PA	25/10	79
LV	140/0–12	95
AO	140/75	96

Questions
1) What is the diagnosis?
2) How would you confirm this diagnosis?

QUESTION 3

A 42 year old man is admitted with a 3 week history of fever, joint pains and abdominal pain. He also admitted that his fingers had felt numb for the past week. He drinks 50 units of alcohol per week, and smoked 20 cigarettes per day.

On examination, temperature was 38.1°C. Pulse 100 bpm, BP 170/100 mmHg. Heart sounds were normal, JVP not elevated. All peripheral pulses were intact, but the fingertips were white bilaterally, with poor capillary return.

Chest was clear, and abdominal examination revealed mild tenderness in the RUQ, but no liver edge was palpable. Sensation was diminished over all the fingers, but the rest of the neurological examination was normal. Bloods were taken for analysis.

Just before the consultant ward round, he complained of central chest pain, and collapsed. Monitoring showed pulseless VT, and he was successfully cardioverted with a 200J DC shock.

Investigations:
Hb 9.9 g/dL
WCC 16.5×10^9/L
Platelets 540×10^9/L
MCV 92 fl
ESR >100 mm/h
CRP 79
Na 129 mmol/L
K 6.5 mmol/L
Urea 34.2 mmol/L
Creatinine 570 μmol/L
Bilirubin 12 μmol/L
ALT 34 iu/L
ALP 420 iu/L

ECG (post arrest):

ST elevation in II, III and aVF
ST depression in I and aVL. Peaked T waves in the anterior leads

Questions
1) What four treatments should he receive immediately?
2) What is the most likely underlying diagnosis?
3) How would you confirm this?

QUESTION 4

A 59 year old woman presented with a 6 week history of weakness, cough and dyspnoea on exertion. She had lost 2 stones in weight over the last 6 months. There was no history of haemoptysis or sputum production. Her GP had recently started her on Prozac because of low mood and poor appetite. She drank alcohol socially, and smoked 20 cigarettes per day.

On examination, she appeared tanned and rather thin. She had finger clubbing. Pulse 90 bpm regular, BP 150/100 mmHg. JVP not raised, heart sounds normal. There was dullness and reduced breath sounds at the right base, and 3 cm hepatomegaly. Neurological examination demonstrated weakness of the shoulder and hip girdles.

Investigations:
ABGs
pH 7.49
pCO_2 4.1 kPa
pO_2 10.1 kPa
Na 141 mmol/L
K 2.7 mmol/L
Urea 3.1 mmol/L
Creatinine 57 μmol/L
FBC normal
Glucose 9.1 mmol/L

Questions
1) What is the most likely diagnosis?
2) Give four investigations to confirm this?

QUESTION 5

A 32 year old woman with a history of Wegener's granulomatosis presents with 2 days of left iliac fossa pain, fever and reduced urine output. She underwent renal transplantation 3 months ago. She takes azathioprine, cyclosporin A, prednisolone, lansoprazole, fosinopril and fluoxetine. She does not smoke or drink alcohol.

On examination, her temperature was 37.8°C. Pulse 90 bpm reg, BP 160/100 mmHg. JVP was not raised, heart sounds were normal and there was no ankle oedema. Chest examination was normal, and abdominal examination revealed a tender mass, 12 × 5 cm in size, in the left iliac fossa.

Investigations:
Hb 12.7 g/d
WCC 12.4 × 10⁹/L
Platelets 195 × 10⁹/L
Na 131 mmol/L
K 5.7 mmol/L
Urea 23.5 mmol/L
Creatinine 385 μmol/L
Bilirubin 14 μmol/L
ALT 81 iu/L
ALP 120 iu/L
Urinalysis: blood +++, protein +. No organisms or casts seen, no growth
Renal ultrasound showed normal doppler flows, an enlarged graft with normal ureter and bladder

Questions
1) What is the most likely diagnosis?
2) Which two tests would you carry out next?

QUESTION 6

A 23 year old waitress presents with apathy and tremor.

Investigations reveal the following:
Na 140 mmol/L
K 3.1 mmol/L
Bicarbonate 14 mmol/L
AST 55 iu/L
Bilirubin 31 μmol/L

Urinalysis glucose ++

Questions
1) What is the likely diagnosis?
2) Give two investigations to confirm the diagnosis.
3) Suggest three physical signs to look for.

QUESTION 7

A 22 year old secretary presents with faintness, sweating and shaking, worse in the morning and relieved by chocolate. She has blacked out twice in the last 4 months. She has gained 9 kg in weight over that period. She complains of no abdominal pain, diarrhoea, respiratory or GU symptoms. She has no history of epilepsy or head injury, smokes 20 cigarettes per day, drinks occasional alcohol and takes the oral contraceptive pill.

She appears mildly obese with a BP of 120/70 mmHg and no postural drop. Cardiovascular, respiratory, abdominal and neurological examination are normal.

Investigations:
FBC normal
U + Es normal
LFTs normal
Calcium 3.04 mmol/L
Albumin 36 mmol/L

An 8 h fast was performed, after which she felt sweaty and faint.

Glucose 1.7 mmol/L
Insulin raised
C-peptide raised

Questions
1) What is the likely underlying diagnosis?
2) Name three tests to confirm this?

QUESTION 8

A 30 year old man with longstanding ulcerative colitis presents with acute upper abdominal pain. He has recently returned from a short visit to his parents in Kenya. His ulcerative colitis is quiescent at present. He has no other medical history of note. He took all the correct prophylaxis for travelling. He does not take any regular medications. Examination reveals a tender right upper abdomen. He does not exhibit guarding or rebound tenderness, and his bowel sounds are normal. He has a mild pyrexia of 37.4°C, but cardiac, respiratory and neurological examination are all unremarkable.

Investigations:
Na 135 mmol/L
K 4.5 mmol/L
Urea 8 mmol/L
Creatinine 100 μmol/L
Hb 7.5 g/dL
WCC 10.9 × 10^9/L
Platelets 300 × 10^9/L
ALT 70 iu/L
ALP 300 iu/L
Bilirubin 35 μmol/L

Albumin 34 g/L
Total protein 50 g/L

Questions
1) Name the four most likely causes for the abdominal pain.
2) Which four investigations would you like to do?

QUESTION 9

A 46 year old teacher presents to Accident and Emergency with a 6 h history of fever, dry cough, dyspnoea and muscle pains. This is the third such episode of illness, the last ones being 4 and 8 weeks ago. He is otherwise fit and well and does not smoke. On examination, temperature is 37.9°C. He is not clubbed or cyanosed and no lymph nodes are palpable. The throat is not inflamed. Pulse is 100 bpm, BP 130/70 mmHg. JVP not raised. Respiratory rate 24/min, with bibasal crepitations audible.

Investigations:
Hb 15.5 g/dL
WCC 13.7 × 10^9/L
Platelets 376 × 10^9/L
FEV1 4.0L
FVC 4.4L
Ratio 90%
Kco 65% predicted

pO_2 8.4 kPa
pCO_2 3.5 kPa
pH 7.44

Questions
1) What is the most likely diagnosis?
2) What corroborating test would you do?

QUESTION 10

A 72 year old woman presents with tingling and weakness in her legs. This started a few days ago when she noticed her feet tripping up whilst walking. The weakness has now spread to her thighs and hips over the last 4 days. For the last 12 hours, she has been unable to walk. She had a bout of diarrhoea a week ago, but is usually well. She complains of no cough, sputum, weight loss or abdominal pain. She takes no medication and does not drink alcohol or smoke.

On examination, she is apyrexial. Pulse 70 bpm reg, BP 90/40 mmHg lying, 70/40 mmHg sitting. JVP not raised. Heart sounds are normal with no ankle oedema. Chest and abdominal examination are normal and she has no back tenderness. Sensation is normal in her legs, power in her arms is normal, but power in her hip muscles is 4/5 and only 2/5 at her knees and ankles. Arm reflexes are normal, but leg reflexes are absent. Plantars are normal.

Investigations:
FBC normal
U + Es normal
Calcium 2.21 mmol/L
LFTs normal
Glucose 5.0
CSF: Glucose 4.1, protein 2.1 g/dL, WBC 4, RBC 0. No growth

Questions
1) What is the probable diagnosis?
2) What investigation should be done next to aid in her immediate management?
3) What treatment should she be given?

QUESTION 11

A 50 year old man presents with a history of recurrent pleural effusions, coal worker's pneumoconiosis and recent onset haemoptysis. Past medical history only reveals a mild arthritis which has been put down to osteoarthritis. He denies fever, cough, weight loss or night sweats but does feel he is more short of breath. He also complains of a non-specific rash occurring on his legs 3 weeks ago. He lives with his wife who is well, and he gave up smoking 2 years ago.

Investigations:
Hb 11 g/dL
WCC 8.0 × 10⁹/L
Platelets 190 × 10⁹/L
Na 140 mmol/L
K 5.0 mmol/L
Urea 25 mmol/L
Creatinine 315 μmol/L

ANCA positive
Urinalysis protein ++ blood +++

Questions
1) Name three conditions which may be the cause.
2) What four investigations would you like to perform?

QUESTION 12

A 45 year old man presents with a one week history of dry cough and breathlessness preceded by headache, and accompanied by pain and reduced hearing in the left ear. He had received a 5 day course of amoxycillin.

He appeared pale and had a temperature of 38.2°C. A rash with target lesions was evident on the trunk. He had a respiratory rate of 24/min, bibasal fine crackles and three finger breadth tender hepatomegaly. There was no splenomegaly.

Results:
Hb 7.2 g/dL
MCV 101 fl
WCC 11.5 × 10⁹/L
Platelets 131 × 10⁹/L
ESR 88 mm/h
U + Es normal
Bilirubin 38 μmol/L
ALT 562 iu/L
ALP 160 iu/L
Reticulocytes 4%
Cold agglutinins present
CXR: bibasal patchy shadows

Questions
1) What is the probable diagnosis?
2) What drug would you give?

QUESTION 13

A 23 year old Tunisian man presented with lower left pleuritic chest pain. It was sudden in onset and worsened over the course of a few hours. He felt hot and sweaty, but complained of no cough, sputum or haemoptysis. He had also noticed tenderness of his right lower leg.

His past medical history included a laparotomy for appendicitis aged 17, and a stay in hospital with suspected septic arthritis of the left knee last year. He did not drink or smoke, and was an orphan.

235

On examination, temperature was 38.7°C. Pulse was 110 bpm, BP 130/90 mmHg. Heart sounds were normal, and the chest was clear. Respirations were 30 per minute and shallow. Abdominal and neurological examination were unremarkable. The right shin was red, hot and tender.

Investigations:
Hb 12.5 g/dL
WCC 19.1 × 10⁹/L
Platelets 402 × 10⁹/L
Na 141 mmol/L
K 4.2 mmol/L
Urea 5.4 mmol/L
Creatinine 110 μmol/L
ESR 95 mm/h
CRP 54 mg/L
Rheumatoid factor negative
ANA negative
ECG: sinus tachycardia, 110/min
CXR: small left pleural effusion

Questions
1) What is the most likely diagnosis?
2) What therapy would you institute?

QUESTION 14

A 50 year old woman was admitted to hospital with a 3 month history of arthritis involving her left knee, right ankle and left elbow. She otherwise felt well but gave a history of occasional episodes of bloody diarrhoea. On examination she was mildly jaundiced.

Investigation revealed the following results:
Bilirubin 40 μmol/L
ALP 500 iu/L
AST 30 iu/L
Albumin 35 g/L

X-rays of the affected joints showed minor degenerative changes.

Questions
1) What is the most likely diagnosis?
2) List four possible causes for the abnormal liver function tests.
3) Give three investigations to confirm your diagnosis.

QUESTION 15

A 30 year old woman presents with symptoms of anorexia, weight loss, arthralgia and fever continuing for the last 5 days. She has vomited twice, and not opened her bowels for 3 days. Apart from visiting family in Africa a month previously, she gives no other relevant history.

On examination she has a temperature of 39°C. Pulse is 80 bpm regular and blood pressure is 100/70 mmHg. There are no other physical signs.

Investigations:
Na 130 mmol/L
K 3.5 mmol/L
Urea 10 mmol/L
Creatinine 130 μmol/L
Hb 10 g/dL
MCV 80 fl
WCC 2.5 × 10⁹/L
Platelets 120 × 10⁹/L
ESR 50 mmHg
PT 18 s
APTT 50 s

Questions
1) Which two tests would be most useful in establishing the diagnosis?
2) What is the most likely diagnosis?
3) How would you treat this?

QUESTION 16

A 30 year old woman presents with headaches occurring in the morning of several weeks' duration. More recently she has noticed intermittent blurring of vision.

On examination she is 96 kg, and has bilateral papilloedema. CT of the head is reported as being normal.

Questions
1) What is the likely diagnosis?
2) What three tests would you perform to establish the diagnosis and assess its severity?
3) Give two initial treatments.

QUESTION 17

A 50 year old man was admitted with a 6 day history of fever and shortness of breath. He had a history of myocardial infarction 2 years ago. He also gave a history of recent travel to Turkey.

On examination he was pyrexial at 38.2°C, pulse 104 bpm. Blood pressure was 110/75 mmHg. The JVP was elevated 5 cm, apex beat displaced with a loud pansystolic murmur heard loudest at the apex. Respiratory examination revealed bibasal crackles and he had ankle oedema.

Investigations:
Hb 10 g/dL
MCV 82 fl
WBC $16 \times 10^9/L$
Platelets $450 \times 10^9/L$

Na 135 mmol/L
K 4.1 mmol/L
Urea 13 mmol/L
Creatinine 180 μmol/L
LFTs normal
Urinalysis: blood ++, protein +++

ECG shows sinus rhythm with Q waves in the anterior leads.

Questions
1) Give the four most important investigations.
2) What is the most likely diagnosis?

QUESTION 18

A 45 year old smoker with late onset asthma presents with cough, and increasing shortness of breath. He also has intermittent chest pains. He feels non-specifically unwell, with anorexia, and weight loss. On examination he has a temperature of 37.8°C and a tachycardia of 110 bpm. He has a blood pressure of 150/100 mmHg. There is a soft pansystolic murmur, widespread polyphonic expiratory wheeze and he has bilateral basal lung crackles. He has a nodular rash on his legs.

Investigations:
Hb 11.0 g/dL
WCC $15 \times 10^9/L$ (80% neutrophils and 5% lymphocytes)
Platelets $180 \times 10^9/L$
ESR 80 mm/h
Na 140 mmol/L
K 4.5 mmol/L

Urea 15 mmol/L
Creatinine 160 μmol/L

Chest X-ray: widespread fluffy shadowing throughout both lung fields.

Questions
1) What is the most likely diagnosis?
2) What three investigations would you perform?
3) What immediate treatment would you instigate?

QUESTION 19

A 49 year old woman is admitted for routine parathyroidectomy. Her father had a neck operation 20 years ago.

Calcium 2.81 mmol/L
PO$_4$ 0.8 mmol/L
Albumin 42 mmol/L
PTH 6.9 nmol/L (normal 0–7.3)
Urinary calcium 0.5 mmol in 24 h

Question
1) Why was the operation cancelled?

QUESTION 20

A 17 year old girl is referred for assessment. She has had sensory loss with pins and needles in both her legs for the last few months, and more recently she has noticed that she is becoming more clumsy and is tripping over more. She has been on fluoxetine for 1 year for depression which has proved rather resistant. She is still low in mood, and is causing trouble at school. She is not sleeping or eating well. There is no other medical history of note.

On examination, she has cerebellar signs in the legs but physical examination is otherwise normal.

Investigations:
MRI head: mild cerebral atrophy.
Lumbar puncture: no oligoclonal bands seen.
    CSF protein 400 mg/L. VDRL negative.
Nerve conduction studies normal.
EEG normal.

Question
1) What is the most likely diagnosis?

237

QUESTION 21

A 22 year old woman presents with right upper quadrant abdominal pain, worse on inspiration. There is no relation to food. She also notes a painful, swollen right knee which has occurred over the last 2 days. She is usually fit and well, takes the oral contraceptive pill, smokes 20 cigarettes per day and drinks 40 units of alcohol per week. She returned from holiday in Spain 2 weeks ago. She denies breathlessness and has no cough.

On examination, she is pyrexial at 37.6°C. There is no jaundice, anaemia or lymphadenopathy. Pulse 90 bpm reg, BP 110/60 mmHg. Heart sounds are normal but there are reduced breath sounds and a rub at the right lung base anterolaterally. Respiratory rate is 16/min. She has tenderness to palpation in her right upper quadrant, with no guarding and no mass or liver palpable. Her right knee is hot, tender and swollen, with very restricted range of movement.

Investigations:
Hb 11.9 g/dL
WCC 12.3×10^9/L
Platelets 180×10^9/L
ESR 92 mm/h
U + Es normal
Bilirubin 28 μmol/L
ALT 135 iu/L
ALP 198 iu/L
Rheumatoid factor negative
ANA negative
Atypical pneumonia serology negative
Blood cultures negative
Joint aspirate 22 000 neutrophils/mL, no growth
CXR: Small right sided pleural effusion
Joint X-ray normal

Questions
1) What is the most likely diagnosis?
2) What investigation would you do to confirm this?

QUESTION 22

A 10 year old boy presents with persistent offensive diarrhoea with abdominal pains following a holiday abroad with his parents who were asymptomatic. He otherwise felt well, with a good appetite. The stools were pale, and bulky. Past medical history includes recurrent sinusitis, and measles as an infant.

On examination he was small for his age. He had no clubbing, jaundice, anaemia, or lymphadenopathy. Respiratory examination revealed a polyphonic wheeze and crackles in his left mid zone and right base. Abdominal examination revealed a palpable loaded colon in the right iliac fossa, but no organomegaly.

Investigations:
Na 137 mmol/L
K 4.2 mmol/L
Urea 5 mmol/L
Creatinine 90 μmol/L
Hb 11 g/dL
WBC 9.5×10^9/L
Platelets 350×10^9/L
Bilirubin 17 μmol/L
Calcium 2.10 mmol/L
Albumin 24 g/L
Total protein 71 g/L
Iron 16 μmol/L
TIBC 46 μmol/L
Vitamin B_{12} 250 pg/mL
Folate 1.9 μg/L

Chest X-ray: atelectasis both bases.
Abdominal plain X-ray: faecal loading in the colon.

Questions
1) What is the most likely diagnosis?
2) Name two investigations to confirm your diagnosis.

QUESTION 23

A 40 year old woman presents with a 4 month history of difficulty getting up from sitting and climbing stairs. She has also noticed aching in her arms and legs. She has a history of hypothyroidism and for this she takes thyroxine. She has had some arthritis in her hands for the past 6 months and a rash across her knuckles.

Results:
Hb 10.2 g/dL
WBC 18.0×10^9/L (Neutrophils 85%, lymphocytes 13%)

Platelets 300×10^9/L
ESR 50 mm/h
Bilirubin 5 μmol/L
Albumin 35 g/L
Total protein 80 g/L
AST 90 iu/L
ALP 120 iu/L
Free T4 80 nmol/L

Muscle biopsy normal

EMG: short polyphasic potentials, with
spontaneous fibrillation

Questions
1) What is the diagnosis?
2) What three further investigations would you
perform to confirm the diagnosis?

QUESTION 24

A 40 year old woman with longstanding
seropositive arthritis returns to rheumatology
outpatients with progressive shortness of breath.
On examination, she is cyanosed, and has
widespread crackles throughout her lung
fields.

Lung function shows:
FVC 2.0 L (predicted 2.4–3.6 L)
FEV_1 1.8 L (predicted 1.8–2.8 L)
FEV_1/FVC 90%
TLC 2.5 L (predicted 5.0–7.5 L)
Kco 65% expected

Questions
1) What is the diagnosis?
2) How would you confirm this?

QUESTION 25

A 45 year old man presents with a history of
lethargy. His only past medical history is of
irritable bowel and an episode of pneumonia
6 months ago. As a businessman, he has spent
much time abroad, including the Far East and
Africa. The reason for attending his GP is that he
now suffers from pleuritic chest pains, and has
developed a cough. On examination he has fever
of 38.5°C, cervical and axillary
lymphadenopathy and he has left-sided crackles
in his chest. Abdominal examination reveals a
large liver and spleen. He is a heavy drinker, and
smokes 20 cigarettes per day.

Initial blood tests show:
Hb 8.0 g/dL
WCC 35×10^9/L (60% neutrophils, 10%
metamyelocytes, 25% myelocytes, 1%
promyelocytes, 2% nucleated red cells)
Platelets 30×10^9

Questions
1) Give three possible diagnoses.
2) What two tests would you like to perform
first?

QUESTION 26

A 78 year old woman with a history of epilepsy
following a stroke 3 years ago presents with
pain and weakness in her legs and
shoulders.

Investigations:
Na 136 mmol/L
K 4.1 mmol/L
Urea 6.8 mmol/L
Creatinine 121 μmol/L
Calcium 2.04 mmol/L
Albumin 39 g/L
PO_4 0.66 mmol/L
Bilirubin 22 μmol/L
ALT 71 iu/L
ALP 277 iu/L
PTH 16.0 nmol/L
ESR 21 mm/h

Questions
1) What is the probable diagnosis?
2) What are the most likely causes for this?

QUESTION 27

A 71 year old woman presented with headaches
and blurred vision.

Results:
Hb 9.2 g/dL
MCV 84 fl
WCC 3.2×10^9/L
Platelets 104×10^9/L
ESR 190 mm/h
Na 142 mmol/L

K 4.4 mmol/L
Urea 5.9 mmol/L
Creatinine 90 μmol/L
Protein 97 g/L
Albumin 34 g/L
Calcium 2.26 mmol/L
Urinalysis: protein +++, blood –

Questions

1) What is the probable diagnosis?
2) How would you treat her headaches and blurred vision?

QUESTION 28

A 54 year old accountant presents to Accident and Emergency with haematemesis and melaena. She gives a 4 month history of upper abdominal discomfort, and has recently been to her GP complaining of a persistent itch. She also complains that her eyes seem dry and sore recently. She gives no history of indigestion, drinks seven units of alcohol per week and has never received a blood transfusion. She has taken thyroxine for 5 years, but takes no other medication.

On examination, her pulse is 120 bpm and regular, BP 85/50 mmHg. Prominent xanthelasma are present. No palmar erythema or spider naevi are noted. She appears to be clubbed, but chest examination is unremarkable. A 4 cm smooth liver edge plus 3 cm spleen tip are palpable in the abdomen; pr examination confirms melaena.

Investigations:
Hb 7.1 g/dL
WCC 13.5 × 10⁹/L
Platelets 540 × 10⁹/L
Na 138 mmol/L
K 4.5 mmol/L
Urea 12 mmol/L
Creatinine 67 μmol/L
Cholesterol 8.7 mmol/L
Protein 81 g/L
Albumin 33 g/L
Bilirubin 28 μmol/L
ALT 41 iu/L
ALP 895 iu/L
INR 1.1
APTTR 1.0

Questions

1) What is the most likely diagnosis?
2) Give two tests to confirm the diagnosis?
3) What are the next three steps you would take?

QUESTION 29

A 59 year old farmer presents with tiredness, loose, offensive stools and 10 kg weight loss over the last 2 years. He describes no rectal bleeding. He has noted some bloating of his abdomen, and also on direct questioning complains of a dry cough and pains in his knees and elbows. He takes no medication and has no past history of illness. He drinks 2 pints of beer per week and does not smoke.

On examination, his temperature is 37.6°C. Pulse 72 bpm reg, BP 95/60 mmHg. He appears suntanned, and several firm lumps are palpable in the supraclavicular area bilaterally. No oral ulcers are noted. JVP not raised. Heart sounds 1 + 2 are heard with a 3/6 PSM at the apex. His ankles are not swollen. Chest was clear. Abdominal examination revealed no palpable liver or spleen; a non-pulsatile mass was palpable in the midline. PR revealed a pale, offensive stool. Neurological examination revealed an abbreviated mental test score of 7 out of 10, but no focal signs. The right knee was mildly swollen and tender.

Investigations:
Hb 10.1 g/dL
WCC 11.6 × 10⁹/L
Platelets 209 × 10⁹/L
Na 138 mmol/L
K 3.4 mmol/L
Urea 2.4 mmol/L
Creatinine 89 μmol/L
Calcium 2.04 mmol/L
Albumin 28 g/L
INR 1.5
Bilirubin 14 μmol/L
ALT 34 iu/L
ALP 199 iu/L
ESR 86 mm/h
CRP 41 mg/L
Faecal fat collection: 21g in 24 h

Questions
1) What is the most likely diagnosis?
2) Name two tests to confirm the diagnosis?

QUESTION 30

A 32 year old Irish woman presents with 9 months of bloating and abdominal cramps. She has offensive, loose stools which are free of blood. She complains of feeling tired and breathless, and has lost 6 kg in weight. She is usually well, and had her fifth child 18 months ago. She takes no medications, does not drink or smoke, and has not been abroad in the recent past.

On examination, she appears pale. Pulse 70 bpm reg, BP 110/70 mmHg with no postural drop. Heart sounds, chest and abdominal examination were normal, as was neurological examination.

Investigations:
Hb 9.4 g/dL
MCV 87 fl
WCC 6.1×10^9/L
Platelets 189×10^9/L
Na 144 mmol/L
K 3.6 mmol/L
Urea 2.7 mmol/L
Creatinine 51 μmol/L
Bilirubin 10 μmol/L
ALT 30 iu/L
ALP 141 iu/L
Calcium 2.10 mmol/L
Albumin 29 g/L
PO_4 0.68 mmol/L
Glucose 4.8 mmol/L
INR 1.5
Blood film: Pencil cells, dimorphic RBCs, with a few Howell-Jolly bodies and some hypersegmented neutrophils

Questions
1) What is the most likely diagnosis?
2) What two investigations would you do to confirm the diagnosis?

QUESTION 31

A 34 year old man presents with a history of dizzy spells. He attends A&E following an episode of dizziness and breathlessness when shopping that almost made him black out. He reports no previous illnesses, but admits on direct questioning to a dry cough and passing a lot of urine recently.

On examination, pulse 40 bpm, regular. BP 100/60 mmHg. He is apyrexial with no lymphadenopathy. The rest of the examination is unremarkable.

Investigations:
Hb 14.6 g/dL
WCC 8.1×10^9/L
Platelets 421×10^9/L
Na 140 mmol/L
K 4.0 mmol/L
Urea 4.1 mmol/L
Creatinine 79 μmol/L
Glucose 5.1 mmol/L
Calcium 2.79 mmol/L
Albumin 38 g/L

ECG: Complete heart block with junctional escape
CXR: Bilateral hilar prominences. Lung fields clear

Tuberculin test: Negative

Questions
1) What is the diagnosis?
2) Which three further investigations would help confirm the diagnosis?

QUESTION 32

An 80 year old man is referred with a history of confusion. He has been living alone, and was found by neighbours in a state of self-neglect and smelling of urine. He is diabetic, hypertensive and has emphysema. He still smokes 20 cigarettes a day but does not drink alcohol. His medications include gliclazide, bendrofluazide and lactulose. On examination, he has a mental test score of 5/30. He is apyrexial, and has a resting heart rate of 80 bpm in atrial fibrillation. His blood pressure is 150/80 mmHg. Respiratory and abdominal examinations are normal. Neurological examination reveals a fine intention tremor. Tone, power, reflexes and coordination are all normal in the arms, but there is hyper-reflexia, increased tone and ataxia of the legs. He is unable to walk unaided.

241

Investigations:
Hb 12.0 g/dL
WCC 7.0 × 10⁹/L
Platelets 200 × 10⁹/L
Na 135 mmol/L
K 4.5 mmol/L
Urea 12 mmol/L
Creatinine 140 μmol/L
ESR 20 mm/h
LFTs normal
TSH 2.0 mU/L
CXR normal
Urinalysis: protein +, culture negative

Question
1) What is the likely diagnosis?
2) What two tests would you like to do?
3) How would you treat this patient?

QUESTION 33

A 27 year old man presents with a 6 h history of central abdominal pain and vomiting. He has not had his bowels open for 2 days, but can pass flatus. The pain is constant, but no worse on coughing. He also complains of tingling in both legs. His only previous contact with the medical profession was a 3 month stay in a psychiatric unit for psychosis 5 years ago. He smokes 20 cigarettes per day and had an alcohol binge 2 days ago.

On examination, his temperature was 38.1°C. Pulse 110 bpm, BP 170/100 mmHg. Chest examination was normal, and abdominal examination revealed no tenderness or guarding, normal bowel sounds and no organomegaly. Sensation was reduced in both feet.

As the examination is concluded, the patient has a generalized seizure, which terminates with diazepam.

Investigations:
Na 126 mmol/L
K 3.8 mmol/L
Urea 7.0 mmol/L
Creatinine 77 μmol/L
Bilirubin 4 μmol/L
ALT 51 iu/L
ALP 77 iu/L
Glucose 5.1 mmol/L
Hb 16.4 g/dL

WCC 17.1 × 10⁹/L
Platelets 410 × 10⁹/L

Questions
1) What is the most likely diagnosis?
2) What bedside test could you do to confirm the diagnosis?

QUESTION 34

A 48 year old woman presents with 4 months of nausea and dizzy spells, weight loss and ankle oedema. The dizzy spells are commonly brought on by drinking sherry, which she uses to try and increase her poor appetite. She also complains of vague abdominal discomfort and loose stools. She has a past medical history of anxiety disorder for which she takes diazepam. She does not smoke.

On examination, she had a reddish face. Pulse 90 bpm reg, BP 120/50 mmHg. Her JVP contained giant V waves, heart sounds 1 + 2 with a pansystolic murmur at the left sternal edge. Ankle oedema was present to the mid thigh level. Examination revealed bilateral pleural effusions; a distended abdomen with shifting dullness and a 6 cm pulsatile liver edge.

Questions
1) What is the likely diagnosis?
2) What tests would you carry out to confirm this?

QUESTION 35

A 31 year old woman is seen in outpatients prior to removal of a recently diagnosed phaeochromocytoma.

PFTs
FEV1 4.7 L
FVC 5.5 L
Kco 42% of predicted

Question
1) What is the probable underlying diagnosis?

QUESTION 36

A 20 year old man presents to the surgeons with severe abdominal pain. For several weeks he has had nausea and vomiting, and for the last 2 days he has complained of severe colicky abdominal pain. The only medication he takes is lactulose for constipation. He smokes 20 cigarettes a day, drinks 3 pints of beer a night, and works for his cousin in a paint stripping business.

Investigations:
Hb 9.5 g/dL
MCV 86 fl
WCC 7.0×10^9/L
Platelets 200×10^9/L
Chest X-ray normal
Abdominal X-ray normal
ECG normal
Urinalysis: glucose ++, protein +, ALA positive, coproporphyrin positive

Question
1) What is the diagnosis?

QUESTION 37

A 50 year old man with longstanding asthma presents with worsening symptoms including fever and productive cough.

Investigations show:
Hb 13.0 g/dL
WCC 10.9×10^9/L (neutrophils 70%, lymphocytes 15%)
Platelets 300×10^9/L
ESR 60 mm/h
Chest X-ray: bilateral mid zone shadows

Questions
1) What is the most likely diagnosis and why?
2) Name two other conditions you would like to rule out and give an investigation to do this.

QUESTION 38

A patient presents with shortness of breath. The data from his cardiac catheter is given below.

	Pressure	Saturation
IVC	20	50%
High RA	26	60%
Low RA	26	56%
RV	100/20	57%
PA	100/30	56%
LV	100/10	70%
Ao	105/80	70%

Question
1) What is the diagnosis?

QUESTION 39

A 25 year old man presents to the Accident and Emergency department with severe loin pain.

Blood tests show:
Na 140 mmol/L
K 3.1 mmol/L
Urea 4.5 mmol/L
Creatinine 100 μmol/L
Chloride 115 mmol/L
Bicarbonate 14 mmol/L

Question
1) What is the diagnosis?

QUESTION 40

A 58 year old woman presented with tiredness, breathlessness and numbness in her feet. Her symptoms had come on gradually over the last year. She had been well for 7 years following a cholecystectomy, which was complicated by an episode of small bowel obstruction 3 weeks post-operatively which required surgical intervention.

On examination, her temperature was 37.7°C. She looked pale. No icterus or lymphadenopathy was noted. Pulse 80 bpm reg, BP 130/60 mmHg. Chest was clear, abdomen soft and non-tender. The spleen was just palpable. She had paraesthesia below the knees, absent ankle reflexes and extensor plantar response.

Investigations:
Hb 7.4 g/dL
WCC 2.3×10^9/L
Platelets 86×10^9/L
MCV 112 fl
Reticulocytes 1%
Bilirubin 41 μmol/L
ALT 18 iu/L
ALP 92 iu/L

Questions
1) What is the most likely diagnosis?
2) What three tests would you do to confirm the diagnosis?

QUESTION 41

A 60 year old man presents with a 9 month history of abdominal pains and loose stools. He has noted 13 kg of weight loss over the past year. The patient also notes that his stool is offensive and tends to float in the pan.

Initial investigation shows
Hb 13.0 g/dL
WCC 7.4×10^9/L
Platelets 250×10^9/L
U&Es normal
3 day faecal fat excretion: 18 g/day

Questions
1) Give three possible diagnoses.
2) Give three investigations to provide the diagnosis.

QUESTION 42

A 76 year old man is admitted with left-sided weakness which had become apparent over the last 24 h. One week prior to admission, he had sustained a fall in the kitchen with transient loss of consciousness. Past medical history included hypertension and atrial fibrillation. No record of his medications was available.

On examination, he was apyrexial. No anaemia, clubbing or jaundice noted. Pulse was 80 irregular. BP 190/100. Cardiovascular and respiratory examination was normal. Neurologically, GCS was 14, with reduced power in the left arm and leg. Both plantars were downgoing. There was no papilloedema, and cranial nerve examination was normal.

Investigations:
Na 129 mmol/L
K 3.2 mmol/L
Urea 6.1 mmol/L
Creatinine 90 μmol/L
Glucose 8.1 mmol/L
FBC normal
INR 2.7
Bilirubin 14 μmol/L
ALT 20 iu/L
ALP 81 iu/L
ECG AF, 90/min. Normal ST segments
CXR shows cardiomegaly

Several hours later, he sustained a generalized seizure on the ward

Question
1) What is the likely diagnosis?

QUESTION 43

A 60 year old lady presents with a progressive history of grumbling fever, weight loss, arthralgia and exertional dyspnoea. She has been previously well, except for long-standing hypertension and a small TIA 2 months previously.

Examination reveals a fever of 37.8°C, and an unwell looking woman. She has a resting tachycardia. Blood pressure is 150/90 mmHg. She has a soft late systolic murmur. Chest and abdominal examinations are normal.

Investigations:
Hb 10.0 g/dL
WCC 12×10^9/L
Platelets 200×10^9/L
ESR 120 mm/h
Na 145 mmol/L
K 4.0 mmol/L
Urea 13.0 mmol/L
Creatinine 150 mmol/L
Urinalysis blood +, protein +
Blood cultures negative
Chest X-ray normal
ANCA, ANA negative

Questions
1) Suggest two possible diagnoses.
2) What is your investigation of choice to establish the diagnosis?

QUESTION 44

A 30 year old Asian man returns from a 4 week trip abroad visiting family. Two weeks after arriving home, he notices a lump on the side of his neck. He presents to his GP who notes that he has lymphadenopathy of the left neck and left axilla. The patient reports feeling somewhat feverish, over the last few weeks. He smokes 20 cigarettes per day and has a chronic dry cough, but otherwise has no other medical problems.

Initial investigation shows:

Hb 12.0 g/dL
WCC 9.2 × 10⁹/L
Platelets 200 × 10⁹/L
ESR 35 mm/h
Na 135 mmol/L
K 4.0 mmol/L
Urea 8.0 mmol/L
Creatinine 100 μmol/L

Question
1) Name three diagnoses which should be excluded initially.
2) What four further investigations should you perform?

QUESTION 45

A 28 year old woman presents with high fever, rigors, vomiting and diarrhoea for one day. On examination, she appears confused, with a widespread blanching macular rash. Pulse 120 reg, BP 75/40. Temp 39.2°C. Chest clear, abdomen soft. PV examination reveals a bloodstained tampon. There is no neck stiffness or photophobia.

Investigations:
Na 128 mmol/L
K 6.1 mmol/L
Urea 22.7 mmol/L
Creatinine 540 μmol/L
Glucose 4.3 mmol/L
CK 1340 iu/L
Hb 12.1 g/dL
WCC 15.4 × 10⁹/L
Platelets 81 × 10⁹/L
Urinary βHCG negative

Questions
1) What is the likely diagnosis?
2) What three therapeutic manoeuvres would you perform next?

QUESTION 46

A 54 year old woman, diagnosed with Raynaud's syndrome 4 years previously presents with a 4 week history of headaches and tiredness. She is otherwise well, takes nifedipine in the winter, and on systems review complains of mild dysphagia and stiff fingers and wrists.

On examination, pulse is 70 bpm reg, BP 190/110 mmHg. Heart sounds are normal, there are fine paninspiratory crackles at both lung bases, and abdominal examination is normal.

Investigations:
Hb 10.2 g/dL
WCC 4.1 × 10⁹/L
Platelets 180 × 10⁹/L
MCV 85 fl
Na 130 mmol/L
K 5.9 mmol/L
Urea 40.7 mmol/L
Creatinine 604 μmol/L
LFTs normal
Urinalysis protein ++, blood –
ANA 1 : 160
dsDNA negative

Lung function:
FEV1 2.8 L
FVC 3.2 L
Ratio 88%
Kco 70% of predicted

Questions
1) What is the probable underlying diagnosis?
2) What confirmatory test may help?
3) What two complications is she suffering from?

QUESTION 47

A 62 year old man presents with right flank discomfort and night sweats.

Hb 18.7 g/dL
WCC 6.8 × 10⁹/L
Platelets 390 × 10⁹/L
ESR 79 mm/h
Na 141 mmol/L
K 3.8 mmol/L
Urea 6.7 mmol/L
Creatinine 117 μmol/L
Bilirubin 8 μmol/L
ALT 13 iu/L
ALP 92 iu/L
Ca 2.84 mmol/L
Alb 41 g/L
Urine: Blood +++, Protein +

Questions
1) What is the most likely diagnosis?
2) What investigation would help confirm this diagnosis?

QUESTION 48

A 20 year old man presents with weakness of his hands and difficulty walking over a period of several months. He denies any sensory symptoms. He had recurrent chest infections as a child but no recent medical problems. He smokes 20 cigarettes per day and drinks roughly 20 units alcohol per week.

On examination, he looks rather wasted. He has weakness in his hand and wrist flexors and he has a bilateral foot drop. Reflexes are reduced. There is no sensory loss.

Investigations:
Creatine kinase: 150 iu/L
ECG: long PR interval and RBBB
EMG: repetitive single motor unit potentials on voluntary contraction, and low amplitude polyphasic motor unit potentials.

Question
1) What is the diagnosis?

QUESTION 49

A 50 year old woman presents with a few months of weight gain and lethargy. She has recently lost her job because she kept falling asleep at work. She also complains of headaches each morning. She has no relevant past medical history. She takes evening primrose oil, but no other regular medication. Her husband who attends with her complains that she snores loudly at night.

On examination, she weighs 100 kg. She has a resting heart rate of 48 bpm, and her blood pressure is 160/90 mmHg. Examination is otherwise normal.

Questions
1) What is the most likely diagnosis?
2) What possible complication has occurred?
3) What two investigations would you do to confirm these diagnoses?

QUESTION 50

A 54 year old man presents with 12 h history of dry cough and shortness of breath. He complains of shivering attacks, and has had loose stools for 4 days since returning from a package holiday in Spain. He is usually fit and well, takes no medication and admits to smoking ten cigarettes per day.

On examination, T = 39.4°C. Pulse is 80/min, BP 90/60. JVP not raised. No ankle oedema. RR = 30/min, with dullness at the left lung base and a few bibasal crepitations. The abdomen is soft and non-tender; pr examination reveals liquid stool with no blood.

Investigations:
Hb 14.0 g/dL
WCC 9.0×10^9/L
Platelets 334×10^9/L
Na 126 mmol/L
K 3.3 mmol/L
Urea 4.6 mmol/L
Creatinine 84 μmol/L

ABGs on air
pO_2 7.2 kPa
pCO_2 3.4 kPa
pH 7.46

CXR: Left pleural effusion. Bilateral lower zone alveolar shadowing.

Questions
1) What is the most likely diagnosis?
2) What drug would you start him on?

QUESTION 51

A 30 year old woman presents with several years' history of tiredness and muscle cramps. She complains of occasional palpitations on direct questioning, and has a tendency towards constipation.

On examination, pulse 70 bpm reg, BP 100/60 mmHg with no postural drop. Normal pigmentation of skin.

Investigations:
Na 134 mmol/L
K 2.3 mmol/L
Urea 3.1 mmol/L
Creatinine 55 μmol/L

Bicarbonate 35 mmol/L
Glucose 5.7 mmol/L
Urinary Na 78 mmol/L
Urinary K 41 mmol/L
Urinary Cl 30 mmol/L
Urinary calcium 2 mmol/L
Urinary diuretic assay: negative on three samples

Questions

1) What is the likely diagnosis?
2) Name two treatments for this condition.

QUESTION 52

A 74 year old man presents with symptoms of
tiredness and bruising. His GP has done a full
blood count which shows:

Hb 8.0 g/dL
MCV 102 fl
WCC 2.0×10^9/L (neutrophils 50%, lymphocytes
40%, Pelger cells seen)
Platelets 50×10^9/L

Questions

1) What is the diagnosis?
2) What investigation should you do to confirm
the diagnosis?

QUESTION 53

A 19 year old woman presents with abdominal
distension and discomfort. Blood tests ordered
by her GP show the following:

Hb 10.8 g/dL
MCV 99 fl
WCC 6.2×10^9/L
Platelets 130×10^9/L
Na 138 mmol/L
K 4.1 mmol/L
Urea 2.2 mmol/L
Creatinine 41 μmol/L
Bilirubin 10 μmol/L
ALT 12 iu/L
ALP 420 iu/L
Amylase 57 iu/L
TSH 1.8 mμ/L

Questions

1) What is the most likely diagnosis?
2) How would you treat this condition?

QUESTION 54

A 20 year old man presents with progressive
clumsiness and loss of balance. He has not
noticed any sensory or visual disturbances. His
mother died when he was 5 years old and had
similar symptoms.

Examination shows nystagmus and ataxia. He
has reduced reflexes in his knees and ankles and
upgoing plantar reflexes. There is some wasting
of his quadriceps but muscle power is normal.

He has a kyphoscoliosis, but cardiac,
respiratory and abdominal examinations are
normal.

Investigations:
U + Es normal
FBC normal
Glucose 10.5 mmol/L

Question

What is the diagnosis?

QUESTION 55

A 28 year old man presents with a 2 day history
of headache and abdominal pain. He also feels
shivery and his muscles and joints ache. He is
normally well apart from well controlled
diabetes, for which he takes twice daily mixed
insulin. He smokes five cigarettes per day, drinks
alcohol occasionally and works as a windsurfing
instructor. He has not been abroad for 2 years.
He complains of no bowel symptoms except for
two loose stools the day before. He has no
respiratory or GU symptoms.

On examination, he is febrile at 39.1°C. He is
not jaundiced and has no lymphadenopathy.
Pulse 110 bpm reg, BP 115/70 mmHg. Heart
sounds are normal as is chest examination.
Abdominal examination reveals 5 cm tender
hepatomegaly. He has melaena on rectal
examination. He has mild photophobia, a stiff
neck and a macular rash on his trunk.
Neurological examination is normal.

Investigations:
Hb 9.4 g/dL
WCC 29.7×10^9/L
Platelets 115×10^9/L
Na 128 mmol/L

K 5.4 mmol/L
Urea 20.1 mmol/L
Creatinine 131 μmol/L
Bilirubin 41 μmol/L
ALT 50 iu/L
ALP 136 iu/L
Glucose 5.0 mmol/L
LDH 970 iu/L
INR 1.3
APTTR 1.2
Haptoglobins absent
CSF: 24 WCC (90% lymphocytes), protein
0.71 g/L, glucose 4.1 mmol/L

Questions
1) What is the most likely diagnosis?
2) What two investigations could confirm the diagnosis?

QUESTION 56

A 50 year old business man presents to rheumatology clinic with increasing pain and swelling of his knee for the last few months. He has recently returned from a business trip abroad. He drinks 3 pints of beer per day. He smokes 40 cigarettes per day.

On examination, he is tanned, and well looking. He has crepitus in both knees. He also has mild hepatomegaly.

Investigations:
Hb 13.0 g/dL
WCC 4.9 × 10⁹/L
Platelets 300 × 10⁹/L
Na 135 mmol/L
K 4.0 mmol/L
Urea 7.0 mmol/L
Creatinine 60 μmol/L
Urinalysis glucose ++

Questions
1) What is the likely single diagnosis?
2) What one investigation would confirm this diagnosis?

QUESTION 57

A 40 year old man presents to A&E with chest pain and shortness of breath. He has had a dry cough for several weeks. He is unkempt, and smells of alcohol and has no fixed abode. He is 6ft tall, and weighs 60 kg. He has a temperature of 37.4°C. He has a few respiratory crackles in the left lung, but the right chest shows reduced breath sounds and increased resonance. He has hepatomegaly and splenomegaly. Oxygen saturation on air is 84%.

Initial investigations:
Hb 10.5 g/dL
WCC 10.9 × 10⁹/L
Platelets 160 × 10⁹/L
Na 145 mmol/L
K 4.0 mmol/L
Urea 10.5 mmol/L
Creatinine 125 μmol/L
AST 60 iu/L
ALP 250 iu/L
Bilirubin 30 μmol/L
Albumin 30 g/L

Chest X-ray:
Right sided pneumothorax. Fibrotic changes of left upper zone, with some calcified nodules.
Blood cultures negative.

Questions
1) What is the most likely diagnosis?
2) What investigation would you do to confirm this diagnosis?
3) Give one immediate and one long-term treatment for this patient.

QUESTION 58

A 50 year old woman presents to rheumatology clinic with a polyarthritis. This has been causing symptoms for several months now, and the GP has been treating her with non-steroidal anti-inflammatory drugs. She has recently recovered from a cold, and she still has a hoarse voice, inflamed eyes and a chronically inflamed nose. She also wears bilateral hearing aids. Physical examination is otherwise unremarkable apart from some knee joint stiffness.

Investigations:
FBC and U + Es normal
Rheumatoid factor negative
ANCA negative
Knee X-rays normal
ECG: 1st degree heart block

Questions

1) What is the possible diagnosis?
2) How would you confirm this diagnosis?

QUESTION 59

A pregnant 35 year old woman attends for her routine 30 week check up. She is feeling well. Her blood pressure is 140/90. Urinalysis shows glucose ++, protein +. There is nothing abnormal to note on physical examination. 2 weeks later, she presents to A&E fitting. Blood pressure is 170/110 mmHg.

Initial investigations show:
Hb 15.0 g/dL
WCC 10.0 × 10⁹/L
Platelets 50 × 10⁹/L
Na 135 mmol/L
K 3.5 mmol/L
Urea 8.8 mmol/L
Creatinine 130 μmol/L
Uric acid 0.9 mmol/L
PT 20 s
APTT 55 s

Questions

1) What is the diagnosis?
2) What three immediate steps would you take?

QUESTION 60

A 70 year old man is admitted having had a fall. He has noticed becoming increasingly clumsy over the last few weeks. His past history includes epilepsy and hiatus hernia. Cimetidine has recently been added to his medications by his GP. He is a long-term smoker of 20 cigarettes a day, and drinks alcohol regularly.
Examination shows equal and reactive pupils. He is somewhat drowsy but is apyrexial and has a heart rate of 56 bpm with a blood pressure of 120/60 mmHg. Cardiac, respiratory and abdominal examination are otherwise normal. He has horizontal nystagmus with dysarthria and limb ataxia. He demonstrates hyperreflexia with bilateral ankle clonus.

Questions

1) Suggest the most likely diagnosis?
2) What single investigation would you do to confirm this?

3) How would you treat this patient?

QUESTION 61

A 49 year old man is noted to be wheezy and short of breath at pre-clerking clinic prior to his inguinal hernia repair. His brother was diagnosed as having emphysema four years previously. He drinks three pints of beer per week and has never smoked.

Investigations:
ECG normal
CXR basal bullae right and left
Hb 15.8 g/dL
WCC 9.1 × 10⁹/L
Platelets 349 × 10⁹/L
Na 141 mmol/L
K 4.5 mmol/L
Urea 3.3 mmol/L
Creatinine 79 μmol/L
Bilirubin 31 μmol/L
ALT 145 iu/L
ALP 390 iu/L

Questions

1) What is the likely underlying diagnosis?
2) What investigation would confirm your diagnosis?

QUESTION 62

A 31 year old fashion advertising executive presented to her GP with a 2 month history of tiredness, dating from her recent promotion. She was under a great deal of stress and complained of low mood. She also felt lightheaded on occasions.
On examination, she appeared tanned. Pulse 70 bpm. BP 90/50 mmHg lying, 60/40 mmHg standing. There was no ankle oedema, chest was clear, and abdominal and neurological examination were unremarkable. The thyroid was not palpable.

Investigations:
Hb 14.7 g/dL
WCC 5.3 × 10⁹/L
Platelets 180 × 10⁹/L
Na 122 mmol/L
K 5.9 mmol/L
Urea 10.1 mmol/L

Creatinine 60 μmol/L
BM stick 3.1 mmol/L
Urine: clear

Questions
1) What is the likely diagnosis?
2) What three confirmatory tests would you perform?

QUESTION 63

A 25 year old Greek woman presents on routine antenatal screening with the following results:

Hb 10.5 g/dL
WCC 6.3 × 10⁹/L
Platelets 250 × 10⁹/L
MCV 65 fl
MCH 24 pg

Questions
1) What are the two most likely possibilities?
2) How would you differentiate these?

QUESTION 64

A 49 year old businessman returns from a recent trip to Kenya and presents with fever, malaise, myalgia and abdominal pains. Whilst away he had taken the appropriate antimalarial prophylaxis. On examination, he had a temperature of 40°C. There was no lymphadenopathy, clubbing or jaundice but he was anaemic. He had normal cardiovascular, respiratory and neurological examination. Abdominal examination revealed tenderness in the right upper quadrant.

Investigations:
Hb 8.0 g/dL
WCC 13.0 × 10⁹/L (90% neutrophils)
Platelets 100 × 10⁹/L
Na 128 mmol/L
K 4.3 mmol/L
Urea 15.2 mmol/L
Creatinine 140 μmol/L
Bilirubin 25 μmol/L
AST 60 iu/L
Blood cultures negative
Urine analysis: protein ++ blood +

Questions
1) What is the most likely diagnosis?
2) Which three tests would you perform?
3) What immediate treatment would you give?

QUESTION 65

A 31 year old Indian woman presents with lethargy and dizziness for 2 years. She believed that her husband had put a spell on her. She also noted that her periods had stopped and that she had recently begun to feel thirsty.
  On examination, she had a small goitre. Pulse was 48 bpm regular, BP 90/50 mmHg lying, 65/30 mmHg standing. Chest and abdominal examination were normal.

Investigations:
Hb 9.2 g/dL
WCC 4.1 × 10⁹/L
Platelets 199 × 10⁹/L
MCV 102 fl
Na 129 mmol/L
K 5.8 mmol/L
Urea 8.1 mmol/L
Creatinine 60 μmol/L
Glucose 19.5 mmol/L

Questions
1) What is the likely underlying diagnosis?
2) Give two investigations to confirm the diagnosis.

QUESTION 66

A 24 year old woman presents with collapse preceded by palpitations. Examination shows mild cyanosis, a regular pulse of 68/min, a raised JVP with large V wave, and a pansystolic murmur heard loudest at the left sternal edge. Abdominal examination reveals hepatomegaly, and she has swollen ankles.
  ECG shows a PR interval of 0.08 s with a delta wave.

Questions
1) What is the diagnosis?
2) How would you confirm your diagnosis?

QUESTION 67

A 63 year old man presents with sudden onset pain in his back which came on whilst he was opening a window. He complains of no weakness or numbness in his legs; bowel and bladder function are normal. He suffered a myocardial infarction 7 years ago, is known to be hypertensive and stopped smoking 7 years ago. He drinks 30 units of alcohol per week. He takes aspirin, a beta blocker and a thiazide diuretic. He complains of no respiratory symptoms, but has been feeling tired for the last 3 months.

On examination, he is apyrexial but in some pain. Pulse 60 bpm reg, BP 140/80 mmHg, JVP not raised, heart sounds are normal. Chest and abdominal examination are normal. There is no neurological deficit in the limbs. Spinal examination reveals marked tenderness at the T6 level.

Investigations:
Hb 10.9 g/dL
MCV 86 fl
WCC 13.1×10^9/L
Platelets 423×10^9/L
Na 141 mmol/L
K 3.3 mmol/L
Urea 12.1 mmol/L
Creatinine 151 μmol/L
Calcium 2.81 mmol/L
Albumin 36 g/L
ESR 95 mm/h
CXR normal
Thoracic spine X-rays show a wedge fracture at T6

Questions
1) What is the most likely diagnosis?
2) What four investigations would you do to confirm the diagnosis?

QUESTION 68

A 40 year old woman presents with acute abdominal pain. Examination reveals tender hepatomegaly and ascites. She denies excessive alcohol ingestion. She takes no regular medications except the contraceptive pill, and occasional analgesia for back pain.

Investigations:
ALT 60 iu/L
Bilirubin 40 μmol/L
Total protein 40 g/L

Albumin 36 g/L
ALP 300 iu/L
HBs Ag negative
Anti-smooth muscle antibodies negative
Anti-mitochondrial antibodies negative
Rheumatoid factor negative

Questions
1) What is the most likely diagnosis?
2) Name one test to confirm your diagnosis.

QUESTION 69

A 75 year old man, who is rather hard of hearing, presents with several months of increasing pain in both legs.

Investigations:
Hb 13.4 g/dL
WCC 5.1×10^9/L
Platelets 261×10^9/L
ESR 11 mm/h
Na 141 mmol/L
K 3.6 mmol/L
Urea 7.4 mmol/L
Creatinine 135 μmol/L
Bilirubin 6 μmol/L
ALT 18 iu/L
ALP 590 iu/L
Calcium 2.47 mmol/L
Albumin 37 g/L
Vitamin D normal
PSA 6 ng/L

Questions
1) What is the most likely diagnosis?
2) Name two confirmatory tests

QUESTION 70

A 28 year old woman, 34 weeks pregnant, was admitted following an episode of weakness in her left arm and leg. She had been complaining of headaches for a few days and had noticed some swelling of her ankles. Past medical history included an episode of psychosis for which she was an inpatient on a psychiatric ward 4 years ago, and a history of epilepsy as a child. She had had no fits since the age of 10 years and took no medications.

Whilst being examined, she had a generalized seizure, which terminated spontaneously. Examination revealed a GCS of 9, pulse 90 bpm, BP 160/110 mmHg. Chest was clear, abdomen was unremarkable. Areas of bruising were noted over her back, shoulders and thighs. She had reduced power on the left, with extensor plantars bilaterally.

Investigations:
Hb 9.1 g/dL
WCC 18.9 × 10⁹/L
Platelets 34 × 10⁹/L
ESR 57 mm/h
Film: Schistocytes
Na 129 mmol/L
K 5.5 mmol/L
Urea 16.1 mmol/L
Creatinine 230 μmol/L
Bilirubin 57 μmol/L
ALT 23 iu/L
ALP 380 iu/L
INR 1.1
APTTR 1.0
CK 290 iu/L
Urine: Blood ++, Protein +

She was given IV magnesium, platelets and underwent emergency Caesarean section. She remained unwell on the obstetric unit, and a few days later had an episode of dysphasia and right-sided weakness lasting 6 h. CT brain showed an old right parietal infarct.

Questions
1) What is the most likely diagnosis?
2) Name three other conditions in the differential?
3) What investigation could confirm the diagnosis?

QUESTION 71

A 35 year old man presents to his GP with lethargy, tiredness and myalgia. On closer questioning, he admits to intolerance of cold weather, low mood and constipation. Apart from being involved in a car crash 6 months earlier, he otherwise has no past medical history. He takes regular pain killers for the myalgia, and lactulose for the constipation. On examination, he is pale

and has coarse skin. He has thinned frontal hair. His heart rate is 56 bpm, with a blood pressure of 130/80 mmHg lying and 110/75 mmHg standing.

Investigations:
Hb 11.0 g/dL
WCC 6.8 × 10⁹/L
Platelets 190 × 10⁹/L
Na 130 mmol/L
K 4.5 mmol/L
Urea 7.0 mmol/L
Creatinine 100 μmol/L
TSH 1.0 mU/L
T4 40 nmol/L

The GP prescribed thyroxine 50 mcg, once daily. The patient was later found at home collapsed by his wife.

Questions
1) What is the most likely cause of the collapse?
2) What immediate treatment would you instigate?
3) Give five further tests you would perform.

QUESTION 72

A 28 year old man, known to inject heroin intravenously, presents with a purpuric rash over his lower legs.

Investigations:
Hb 10.3 g/dL
WCC 9.1 × 10⁹/L
Platelets 120 × 10⁹/L
ESR 120 mm/h
Na 133 mmol/L
K 4.7 mmol/L
Urea 14.1 mmol/L
Creatinine 180 μmol/L
Bilirubin 19 μmol/L
ALT 318 iu/L
ALP 140 iu/L
IgG 4.1 g/L
IgA 2.7 g/L
IgM 0.1 g/L
Urinalysis shows protein ++++, blood +.
  No Bence-Jones proteins

Questions
1) What is the most likely diagnosis?
2) Which two tests would you do to help confirm the diagnosis?

QUESTION 73

A 32 year old woman presents with sudden shortness of breath. She gives a history of a mild cough over the preceding few months and she had occasional nose bleeds. She had no history of asthma and took no regular medications except occasional paracetamol for 'rheumatics'.

Examination was unremarkable except for a faint macular rash on her legs which she had not noticed before.

Results:
Hb 13.0 g/dL
WBC 10.2×10^9/L
Platelets 400×10^9/L
Na 140 mmol/L
K 5.0 mmol/L
Urea 15.4 mmol/L
Creatinine 190 μmol/L
ESR 80 mm/h
Urinalysis: protein ++ blood +++
Chest X-ray: several nodular shadows in both lung fields

Questions
1) What is the most likely diagnosis?
2) What three investigations would help confirm the diagnosis?

QUESTION 74

A 32 year old man is brought to the A&E department having been found unconscious at home. He lives alone in a rented flat. There are no localizing neurological signs, pupils are reactive and of normal size and there is no sign of trauma.

Investigations:
Na 144 mmol/L
K 3.7 mmol/L
Urea 3.1 mmol/L
Creatinine 60 μmol/L
LFTs normal
Glucose 5.1 mmol/L

ABGs:
pO_2 21 kPa (on 60% O_2)
O_2 sats 67%
pCO_2 3.3 kPa
pH 7.21

Questions
1) What is the most likely diagnosis?

QUESTION 75

The following results were obtained after administering 75 g of glucose in solution to a 63 year old man:

Time	Glucose	GH
0 min	5 mmol/L	12 mcg/L
30 min	8	11
60 min	10	14
90 min	9	11
120 min	6	

Questions
1) What is the diagnosis?
2) What other investigation would help define the disease better?

QUESTION 76

A 40 year old man presented with recurrent diarrhoea of some years' duration which had always been treated effectively by the GP with metronidazole and loperamide. Past history revealed chest infections that required considerable absence from school. He had also been seen once by a local surgeon to treat a perianal abscess.

Examination revealed cervical lymphadenopathy and a palpable spleen.

Results:
Hb 13.5 g/dL
WBC 5.5×10^9/L
Platelets 340×10^9/L
Na 140 mmol/L
K 4.0 mmol/L
Urea 6.5 mmol/L
Creatinine 100 μmol/L
Bilirubin 15 μmol/L
AST 30 iu/L
ALP 150 iu/L
Albumin 40 g/L
Total protein 61 g/L
Rheumatoid factor negative
HIV test negative
Stool culture negative

Questions

1) What is the diagnosis?
2) What four investigations would you do?

QUESTION 77

A 70 year old man presents with collapse to the local hospital. He has recently complained of fever, shortness of breath, and cough productive of yellow sputum. The GP had started erythromycin 5 days ago to cover a presumed chest infection. For the last 2 days he has felt nauseated, and has had rather loose stools. He takes regular aspirin, bendrofluazide and digoxin.

He has a resting heart rate of 56 bpm irregular, and a blood pressure of 110/60 mmHg. Cardiac examination is normal. Chest examination reveals left-sided basal crackles with bronchial breathing.

Investigations:
Na 135 mmol/L
K 3.4 mmol/L
Urea 5.0 mmol/L
Creatinine 110 μmol/L
CXR left lower zone consolidation

ECG shows atrial fibrillation with a rate of 40 bpm. QRS complexes are 120 ms wide. There is widespread ST depression of 2 mm and T wave inversion in the anterior leads.

Whilst on CCU, a short run of non-sustained VT is noted on his cardiac monitor.

Questions

1) What is the most likely cause of the collapse?
2) Give one investigation to support the diagnosis.
3) What management would you suggest?

QUESTION 78

A 40 year old businessman presents with rash. This covers his trunk and arms and includes the palms of his hands. He also complains of headache, arthralgia and feeling non-specifically unwell. On examination, he has a fever of 37.5°C and the rash is macular in nature. He has a generalized lymphadenopathy involving the cervical, axillary and groin lymph nodes. There are no other abnormalities found.

Investigations:
FBC and U + Es normal

LFTs:
AST 60 iu/L
Bilirubin 30 μmol/L
ALP 150 iu/L
Albumin 36 g/L
Total protein 74 g/L

Questions

1) What is the most likely diagnosis?
2) What investigation would confirm your diagnosis?
3) What disease would you like to exclude?
4) What is the treatment?

QUESTION 79

A 42 year old woman presents with a tender swollen left leg. She is usually well, save for occasional abdominal pains and headaches. She has also had several episodes of painless haematuria, which her GP is investigating. Past medical history includes an episode of aplastic anaemia 2 years ago, for which she received blood product support but no bone marrow transplant.

On examination, she is apyrexial. No jaundice, anaemia, clubbing or lymphadenopathy. Cardiovascular and respiratory examination is normal. Abdominal examination reveals a 2 cm liver edge and a 3 cm spleen. Her left leg is swollen to the mid calf with pitting oedema and venous congestion.

Investigations:
Hb 9.6 g/dL
MCV 82 fL
WCC 2.4 × 10^9/L
Platelets 71 × 10^9/L
U + Es normal
INR 1.0
APTTR 1.1
Bilirubin 41 μmol/L
ALT 36 iu/L
ALP 77 iu/L

Questions

1) What is the likely underlying diagnosis and why is her leg swollen?
2) What three tests would you perform?

QUESTION 80

A 70 year old woman presents with headaches and joint pains. She also complains of fatigue, weight loss and low grade pyrexia. She is previously fit apart from mild osteoarthritis, for which she takes regular analgesics.

Investigations:
Hb 11.0 g/dL
WCC 10×10^9/L
Platelets 400×10^9/L
ESR 70 mm/h
CRP 40 mg/L
Bilirubin 15 μmol/L
AST 25 iu/L
ALP 400 iu/L
Creatine kinase 150 iu/L
Temporal artery biopsy negative

Questions
1) What is the most likely diagnosis?
2) What therapy would you instigate?

QUESTION 81

A 25 year old woman is seen in outpatients following the birth of her first child. She has noticed blurring of vision in her left eye, which was associated with pain. Two years ago she had an episode of vertigo which was put down to a labyrinthitis and which resolved spontaneously.

Questions
1) What is the most likely diagnosis?
2) List three investigations to confirm this diagnosis.
3) What therapy would you offer?

QUESTION 82

A 55 year old man presents with severe diarrhoea and abdominal pains. He has lost 2 stone in weight over the last 6 months. He has a long history of Crohn's disease and has had multiple bowel resections for this over the years. Recently he had become so weak that he was confined to bed.

Examination reveals a cachectic man with multiple abdominal scars from previous surgery. There was also marked wasting of the quadriceps muscles with weakness.

Questions
1) Give four causes for the diarrhoea.
2) What are the two most important investigations to confirm the cause of diarrhoea?

QUESTION 83

A 61 year old woman complains of diplopia. This started on the evening of admission; she had felt sick and noted a dry mouth during the day. By the time of admission to hospital, she was feeling generally weak and had difficulty catching her breath.

On examination, she was apyrexial. Pulse 70 bpm, BP 80/50 mmHg. Chest and abdomen unremarkable. Pupils were fixed and dilated, and she was unable to follow a finger. She had bilateral ptosis. Her voice was hoarse and she could whisper only. She was pooling saliva and could not extend her tongue. Power 2/5 in the arms, 4/5 both legs. Reflexes were diminished in the upper limbs. Tone was universally diminished.

Investigations:
Hb 12.2 g/dL
WCC 8.1×10^9/L
Platelets 420×10^9/L
Na 140 mmol/L
K 4.6 mmol/L
Urea 3.1 mmol/L
Creatinine 90 μmol/L
Glucose 4.7 mmol/L
Tensilon test: no response
CSF: Protein 420 mg/L, WCC 2 lymphocytes, glucose 3.7 mmol/L
PFTs: FEV1 = 0.9L, FVC = 1.2L. Ratio 75%

Questions
1) What is the most likely diagnosis?
2) How would you confirm this?
3) What are the next three essential steps in managing this lady?

QUESTION 84

A 31 year old woman presents with a 4 week history of sweats, fever and aching joints. She had felt generally tired and unwell since returning from a trip to Greece. She was normally healthy, took no medications, drank 30 units of alcohol per week, and smoked ten cigarettes per day. She reported 3 kg weight loss since her holiday, no cough or sputum, but found that she was breathless climbing stairs. Her bowels were normal.

On examination, she looked pale. No rashes or lymphadenopathy were noted. T = 37.8°C. Pulse 90 bpm reg. BP 155/90 mmHg. JVP not raised. Heart sounds normal. The right calf was swollen and mildly tender below the knee. Chest examination was normal. The spleen was just palpable in the abdomen. Neurological examination was normal. Both knees, elbows and shoulders were tender to touch, but were not swollen.

Investigations:
Hb 7.7 g/dL
MCV 103 fl
WCC 3.2 × 10⁹/L
Platelets 78 × 10⁹/L
ESR 113 mm/h
CRP 12 mg/L
INR 1.0
APTTR 1.7
Na 129 mmol/L
K 5.1 mmol/L
Urea 17.6 mmol/L
Creatinine 343 μmol/L
Bilirubin 25 μmol/L
ALT 14 iu/L
ALP 93 iu/L
Albumin 29 g/L
Calcium 2.21 mmol/L
CK 40 iu/L
CXR: normal
Urine: blood ++, protein +++

Questions
1) What is the probable underlying diagnosis?
2) Why is her calf swollen?
3) Name three tests that would allow her disease to be defined better?

QUESTION 85

A 15 year old girl who has just returned home to the UK from a holiday visiting family in India presents with a 5 day history of sharp chest pains made worse by inspiration and lying down. She gives a history of recurrent tonsillitis. Examination reveals a fever of 38.0°C, a soft pericardial rub with a systolic murmur. She has a normal respiratory examination, but locomotor examination reveals tender and swollen joints with restricted movements in the right knee and right elbow. Some results are shown.

Hb 12.0 g/dL
WCC 12 × 10⁹/L
Platelets 200 × 10⁹/L
ESR 70 mm/h

Blood cultures negative
CXR normal

ECG shows sinus rhythm with 1st degree heart block.

Questions
1) Name two possible diagnoses.
2) Which is the most likely?
3) What is the initial treatment?

QUESTION 86

A 22 year old man is admitted unconscious and fitting. He has no other medical history of note. On examination he has a temperature of 41°C. He is cyanosed, and has a heart rate of 140 bpm. Initial blood pressure was 80/40 mmHg. Respiratory examination revealed widespread crackles.

Investigations:
Na 130 mmol/L
K 6.5 mmol/L
Urea 25 mmol/L
Creatinine 350 μmol/L
Hb 14.0 g/dL
WCC 10 × 10⁹/L
Platelets 50 × 10⁹/L
Prothrombin time 25 s
APTT 60 s

Questions
1) What is the most likely diagnosis?
2) What complications have occurred?
3) What two further tests would help confirm the diagnosis?
4) What initial treatment would you give?

QUESTION 87

A 34 year old man presents with a 4 week history of headache and lethargy. The headache is worse in the morning. He also complains of blurred vision, double at times. He complains of nausea, but no vomiting.

He is usually well, the only recent illness being an episode 4 years ago with fever, rash and tender glands. This was diagnosed as glandular fever by his GP. His only other complaint is of a 2 month history of loose stools. He has lost 4 kg in weight during this period. He takes no medicines, drinks occasional alcohol and does not smoke. He lives alone and works as a tattoo artist.

On examination, his temperature was 37.4°C. He had 1 cm tender cervical lymph nodes. No rash or jaundice was noted. Pulse was 80 bpm regular, BP 120/60 mmHg. Heart sounds were normal, chest was clear and abdomen was soft and non tender. He had slight blurring of the disk margins bilaterally, mild neck stiffness and a left sixth nerve palsy.

Investigations:
Hb 15.1 g/dL
WCC 6.7 × 10⁹/L
Platelets 290 × 10⁹/L
U + Es, LFTs normal
ESR 21 mm/h
CRP 15 mg/L
CXR normal

Questions
1) What is the differential diagnosis for his headache?
2) What three investigations would you do next?

QUESTION 88

A 40 year old woman presents to accident and emergency with increasing confusion. There is a preceding history of diarrhoea for 2 weeks, and she has recently started vomiting. She also has non-insulin dependent diabetes mellitus, hypertension and depression. Her medications include gliclazide, bendrofluazide, lisinopril and lithium.

On examination she is drowsy and confused but apyrexial. She has a heart rate of 56 bpm with a blood pressure of 90/50 mmHg. Her chest is clear and she has hyperreflexia with increased tone.

Investigations:
Hb 13.0 g/dL
WCC 14 × 10⁹/L
Platelets 200 × 10⁹/L
Na 128 mmol/L
K 2.7 mmol/L
Urea 30 mmol/L
Creatinine 405 μmol/L
Urine analysis: protein +, blood –, glucose –
ECG: sinus bradycardia
Chest X ray normal

Questions
1) What test would you like to do?
2) What immediate treatment would you start?
3) What is the most likely diagnosis?

QUESTION 89

A 20 year old man with nodular sclerosing Hodgkin's lymphoma on cytotoxic chemotherapy is admitted with shortness of breath.

Examination is normal.

Chest X-ray shows bilateral midzone shadowing.

Questions
1) Give three possible causes for the radiographic findings.
2) Name one investigation to elucidate the cause.

QUESTION 90

A 19 year old girl is admitted comatose, having been found at home by her boyfriend, with whom she has argued after a heavy night's drinking. An empty bottle of tablets was found by paramedics in the kitchen.

On examination, she was apyrexial. Pulse 130/min, BP 80/40, JVP not raised. Chest is clear to auscultation, abdomen soft. Pupils are dilated, GCS = 3, extensor plantars bilaterally. No neck stiffness.

Investigations:
Hb 13.1 g/dL
WCC 9.0×10^9/L
Platelets 225×10^9/L
Na 138 mmol/L
K 4.0 mmol/L
Urea 3.0 mmol/L
Creatinine 59 μmol/L
Glucose 4.8 mmol/L
Bilirubin 10 μmol/L
ALT 110 iu/L
ALP 92 iu/L
CK 533 iu/L
Osmolality 310 mosm/kg
ECG: Sinus tachycardia, 130/min
pO_2 18 kPa (on 60% O_2)
pCO_2 3.1 kPa
pH 7.28

Questions
What is the likely diagnosis?

QUESTION 91

A 40 year old man from Kenya who had never smoked cigarettes presented to Accident and Emergency with a persistent cough and haemoptysis for 4 months with no dyspnoea, chest pain or sputum production. A chest radiograph taken for a routine medical 1 year ago is normal. He is on no regular medications. The only risk factor for thrombosis is a flight home 4 months ago.

Examination was unremarkable.

Investigations show:
Hb 13.0 g/dL
WBC 6.9×10^9/L
Platelets 200×10^9/L
Prothrombin time 14 s
CXR normal

Questions
1) Give three possible causes for the haemoptysis.
2) What four investigations should be undertaken to make a diagnosis?

QUESTION 92

A 67 year old woman presents to A & E with dizzy spells. She is normally well, a keen walker who has no previous history of dizziness, chest pain or breathlessness. She last visited her GP 4 weeks ago, who diagnosed Bell's palsy, which has since improved spontaneously. She takes antihistamines for a rash which she first noted 8 weeks ago after returning from holiday.

On examination, she is apyrexial. No rash is noted. Pulse is 40 bpm regular, BP 100/50 mmHg. JVP not raised. Heart sounds are normal, there is no ankle oedema. Chest and abdominal examination are unremarkable. Neurological examination reveals facial and forehead weakness on the right.

Investigations:
Hb 13.4 g/dL
WCC 7.1×10^9/L
Platelets 241×10^9/L
ESR 47 mm/h
U + Es normal
Bilirubin 24 μmol/L
ALT 14 iu/L
ALP 72 iu/L
ECG: Complete heart block with junctional escape at 40 per minute
Chest X-ray is normal

Questions
1) What is the most likely diagnosis?
2) What treatment would you give?

QUESTION 93

A 34 year old woman is referred to clinic for investigation of twitching.

Investigations:
U + Es normal
FBC normal
LFTs normal
CK 261 iu/L
Calcium 1.6 mmol/L
Albumin 38 g/L
PO_4 1.51 mmol/L
Magnesium 0.77 mmol/L
PTH 22 nmol/L
B_{12} + folate normal
INR 1.0
Vitamin D 61 mmol/L
ECG: Prolonged QT interval (520 ms)

Questions
1) What is the diagnosis?
2) What tests would allow the diagnosis to be defined better?

QUESTION 94

A 28 year old woman presents with an 8 week history of fever and night sweats, following a bout of tonsillitis. In addition, she has complained of bilateral wrist swelling and tenderness, shortness of breath, and a transient macular rash over the last 2 weeks.

On examination, her temperature is 39.8°C. Pulse 90 bpm reg, BP 110/50 mmHg. JVP not raised. Normal heart sounds. No rash is evident, but the wrists are tender, red and swollen. Dullness to percussion and reduced breath sounds are evident at the right lung base.

Investigations:
Hb 9.5 g/dL
WCC 16 × 10⁹/L
Platelets 620 × 10⁹/L
ESR 110 mm/h
ASO titre negative
ANA negative
Rheumatoid factor negative
dsDNA negative
Chest X-ray: right pleural effusion

Questions
1) What is the most likely diagnosis?
2) What treatment would you give?

QUESTION 95

A 30 year old man presents to the A&E department with a suspected overdose of unknown tablets with some alcohol. On examination he had a heart rate of 130 bpm, a blood pressure of 180/110 mmHg, and he was tachypnoeic. Respiratory examination revealed bilateral basal crackles. Neurological examination showed dilated and slow reacting pupils, hypotonia, reduced tendon reflexes and flexor plantar responses.

Initial investigations show:
Hb 15.0 g/dL
WCC 20 × 10⁹/L

Platelets 300 × 10⁹/L
Na 148 mmol/L
K 4.8 mmol/L
Urea 10.5 mmol/L
Creatinine 250 μmol/L
Chloride 85 mmol/L
pH 7.12
Bicarbonate 4.0 mmol/L
Glucose 5.0 mmol/L
Paracetamol not detected
Salicylate not detected

Questions
1) What is the diagnosis?
2) What three tests would you like to perform?
3) What is the treatment of choice?

QUESTION 96

A 30 year old woman presents with variable diplopia. She had a flu-like illness 4 weeks ago, but has now recovered. She has rheumatoid arthritis treated with penicillamine, and a past history of hyperthyroidism.

Examination reveals normal eye movements, limb power and reflexes.

Questions
1) What is the likely diagnosis?
2) What else should be considered?
3) Give three investigations.

QUESTION 97

A 22 year old girl presents with a 5 day history of jaundice, abdominal pain and confusion. She was unable to give any further history, but her parents denied previous ill health, medications or depression.

On examination she was apyrexial. Pulse 95/reg, BP 100/50. JVP not raised and chest clear. She was jaundiced, with 5 cm tender hepatomegaly and ascites. Asterixis was present and her GCS was 13/15.

Investigations:
Hb 10.1 g/dL
WCC 11.0 × 10⁹/L
Platelets 186 × 10⁹/L
INR 2.3
ESR >100 mm/h

259

Na 139 mmol/L
K 4.9 mmol/L
Urea 9.1 mmol/L
Creatinine 67 μmol/L
Amylase 44 iu/L
Glucose 3.0 mmol/L
Bilirubin 122 μmol/L
ALT 3565 iu/L
ALP 410 iu/L

Paracetamol levels undetectable
Urinary drug screen negative
Hepatitis A, B, C, E serology negative
EBV serology shows low titres of IgG. IgM
  negative
CMV serology negative
ANA titre 1/160
Anti-smooth muscle antibody titre 1/320
Anti-mitochondrial antibody negative
Caeruloplasmin normal
Urinary copper normal

Question
1) What is the diagnosis?

QUESTION 98

A 64 year old man with a 20 year history of
rheumatoid arthritis presents with tiredness and
shortness of breath. He takes penicillamine for
his arthritis, but has not been under
rheumatological follow up for several years. He
smokes ten cigarettes per day. He has a
symmetrical, deforming polyarthropathy, Several
finger joints are stiff and tender. T 37.2°C, pulse
80 bpm, BP 140/80 mmHg. JVP + 7 cm, heart
sounds normal. Ankle oedema to the mid thighs
was noted. Chest was clear to auscultation, and
the abdomen was distended and dull to
percussion in the flanks. A 4 cm liver edge was
noted, and the spleen tip was palpable.

Investigations:
Hb 8.1 g/dL
WCC 4.8 × 10⁹/L
Platelets 237 × 10⁹/L
ESR 82 mm/h
Na 126 mmol/L
K 5.4 mmol/L
Urea 28.2 mmol/L
Creatinine 465 μmol/L

Albumin 21 g/L
Bilirubin 27 μmol/L
ALT 13 iu/L
ALP 322 iu/L
ECG: 1° block, RBBB plus left axis deviation
CXR: small heart, bilateral small pleural
  effusions
Urine: Protein ++++. Blood +/–

Questions
1) What is the most likely diagnosis?
2) Give one confirmatory test?

QUESTION 99

A 23 year old woman presents with a pulmonary
embolism. Her admission blood results (before
initiation of therapy) are as follows:

Hb 12.3 g/dL
WCC 5.1 × 10⁹/L
Platelets 82 × 10⁹/L
ESR 7 mm/h
INR 1.0
APTTR 1.6
ANA –ve
VDRL +ve
Na 140 mmol/L
K 4.1 mmol/L
Urea 2.3 mmol/L
Creatinine 47 μmol/L

Questions
1) What is the underlying diagnosis?
2) How could you confirm this?

QUESTION 100

A 47 year old farmer presents with a 6 month
history of intermittent back pain, fever and
weight loss of 6 kg. He also complains of
headaches when feeling feverish, along with
occasional abdominal pain and constipation. A
colonoscopy performed 1 month ago was
normal. He is known to be hypertensive, for
which he takes an ACE inhibitor. He lives with
his wife, who is well, denies any extramarital sex
and does not smoke or drink. He admits to no
respiratory or GU symptoms.

On examination, temperature was 37.4°C.
There was no rash or lymphadenopathy. Pulse

was 70 bpm reg, BP 160/90 mmHg. The rest of the cardiovascular and respiratory examination was normal. Abdominal examination revealed a spleen tip, but no hepatomegaly. PR was normal. Neurological examination was normal, and examination of the back revealed diffuse spinal tenderness.

Investigations:
Hb 9.4 g/dL
MCV 87 fl
WCC 4.1×10^9/L with 1.2×10^9/L neutrophils
Platelets 171×10^9/L
ESR 81 mm/h
Fe 8 μmol/L
TIBC 21 μmol/L
U + Es normal

Albumin 33 g/L
Calcium 2.31 mmol/L
Bilirubin 14 μmol/L
ALT 51 iu/L
ALP 107 iu/L
Rheumatoid factor negative
ANA negative
PSA 4 ng/L
CXR normal
U/S abdomen showed enlarged spleen
Spine X-rays normal

Questions
1) What is the most likely diagnosis?
2) Name one differential diagnosis
3) What three investigations would you do next?

ANSWERS TO QUESTIONS

13

QUESTION 1
1) Behçet's disease
2) Crohn's disease, ulcerative colitis, Reiter's disease
3) Colonoscopy or barium studies. Pathergy test is also a possibility

QUESTION 2
1) ASD
2) Transthoracic echocardiogram

QUESTION 3
1) Calcium (chloride or gluconate) and insulin/dextrose infusions, Aspirin and thrombolysis
2) Polyarteritis nodosa
3) Angiography – digital, coronary or mesenteric. ANCA antibodies

QUESTION 4
1) Cushing's syndrome secondary to lung carcinoma
2) Urinary free cortisol, then low dose dexamethasone suppression test, ACTH levels and CT thorax

QUESTION 5
1) Acute rejection of renal transplant
2) Renal biopsy and cyclosporin level

QUESTION 6
1) Wilson's disease
2) Serum caeruloplasmin, liver biopsy for histology and liver copper levels
3) Kayser-Fleischer rings, sunflower cataracts, hepatomegaly, splenomegaly, blue lunulae in nails

QUESTION 7
1) MEN 1 with parathyroid hyperplasia and an insulinoma
2) Pancreatic ultrasound, PTH level, genetic analysis

QUESTION 8
1) Gallstones, cholangitis, atypical pneumonia, sickle cell disease, malaria
2) Blood film, Hb electrophoresis, liver ultrasound and chest X-ray

QUESTION 9
1) Extrinsic allergic alveolitis (in this case from clearing out the birdcage in the classroom)
2) Serum precipitins

QUESTION 10
1) Guillain-Barré syndrome
2) Spirometry for FVC
3) IV immunoglobulin

QUESTION 11
1) Goodpasture's syndrome, Wegener's granulomatosis, Churg-Strauss disease, microscopic polyarteritis
2) Chest X-ray, renal biopsy, anti-GBM antibodies, dsDNA antibodies

QUESTION 12
1) *Mycoplasma* pneumonia
2) A macrolide (e.g. erythromycin) or a tetracycline

QUESTION 13
1) Familial Mediterranean fever
2) Colchicine

QUESTION 14
1) Ulcerative colitis
2) Primary sclerosing cholangitis, pericholangitis, acute hepatitis, autoimmune cholangiopathy
3) Rectal biopsy, double contrast barium enema, liver ultrasound

QUESTION 15
1) Thick and thin blood films and blood cultures for *Salmonella typhi* culture
2) Typhoid fever
3) Ciprofloxacin

QUESTION 16
1) Benign intracranial hypertension
2) Lumbar puncture for CSF analysis and pressure, MRI head to exclude sagittal sinus thrombosis and visual field analysis
3) Weight reduction and carbonic anhydrase inhibitor

QUESTION 17
1) Multiple blood cultures over several hours and from several venepuncture sites, chest X-ray, transoesophageal echocardiography, urine M, C and S
2) Infective endocarditis of the mitral valve

QUESTION 18
1) Churg-Strauss syndrome
2) Renal biopsy, blood cultures to exclude bacterial pneumonia or endocarditis,

echocardiogram to exclude infective
endocarditis
3) Steroids

QUESTION 19
1) The diagnosis is familial hypocalciuric
hypercalcaemia, not hyperparathyroidism,
thus no operation is necessary

QUESTION 20
1) Variant CJD. Multiple sclerosis has
essentially been excluded by the lack of
plaques seen on MRI, normal nerve
conduction, and normal CSF analysis

QUESTION 21
1) Gonococcal infection with perihepatitis
2) High vaginal/endocervical swabs

QUESTION 22
1) Cystic fibrosis
2) Sweat test for sodium concentration, Lundh
test for pancreatic exocrine function

QUESTION 23
1) Dermatomyositis
2) Repeat muscle biopsy, CK, ANA

QUESTION 24
1) Pulmonary fibrosis secondary to rheumatoid
arthritis
2) CT chest, open lung biopsy

QUESTION 25
1) Myeloid leukaemia (acute or chronic),
myelofibrosis, lung cancer with pneumonia,
malaria
2) Bone marrow and trephine, chest X-ray

QUESTION 26
1) Osteomalacia
2) Anticonvulsant therapy, lack of exposure to
sun with age and previous stroke

QUESTION 27
1) Waldenström's macroglobulinaemia
2) Plasmapheresis, followed by an alkylating
agent (melphalan or chlorambucil)

QUESTION 28
1) Primary biliary cirrhosis
2) Antimitochondrial antibody, liver biopsy
3) Fast IV fluids, blood transfusion, urgent upper
GI endoscopy

QUESTION 29
1) Whipple's disease
2) Duodenal biopsy, lymph node biopsy, PCR of
CSF

QUESTION 30
1) Coeliac disease
2) Anti-endomysial antibody, duodenal
biopsy

QUESTION 31
1) Sarcoidosis
2) Bronchoscopy with biopsy, CT chest and
cardiac biopsy

QUESTION 32
1) Normal pressure hydrocephalus
2) Blood glucose, CT head
3) Acetazolamide

QUESTION 33
1) Acute intermittent porphyria
2) Leave a sample of urine to stand in the light;
it should turn dark

QUESTION 34
1) Tricuspid regurgitation and right heart failure
due to carcinoid syndrome
2) Urinary 5 HIAA level, echocardiography,
liver ultrasound +/– CT abdomen, ^{123}I-MIBG
scanning

QUESTION 35
1) Neurofibromatosis

QUESTION 36
1) Lead poisoning

QUESTION 37
1) ABPA because of the history of asthma, mid
zone consolidation and the likelihood of
eosinophilia
2) Churg-Strauss syndrome, and sarcoidosis.
Lung biopsy would rule out both Churg-
Strauss syndrome and sarcoidosis (a positive
skin prick test would help confirm the
diagnosis of ABPA)

QUESTION 38
1) Eisenmenger's syndrome secondary to an
ASD

QUESTION 39
1) Renal tubular acidosis type I

QUESTION 40
1) Vitamin B_{12} deficiency secondary to terminal ileal resection
2) Folate level, B_{12} level and Schilling test

QUESTION 41
1) Chronic pancreatitis, coeliac disease, pancreatic carcinoma
2) Plain film abdominal X-ray, CT abdomen, endoscopy and duodenal biopsy

QUESTION 42
1) Subdural haemorrhage

QUESTION 43
1) Atrial myxoma and infective endocarditis
2) Transoesophageal echocardiography

QUESTION 44
1) Lymphoma, tuberculosis, metastatic malignancy
2) Chest X-ray, lymph node biopsy, CT chest, abdomen, sputum sample for acid fast bacilli

QUESTION 45
1) Toxic shock syndrome (due to infected tampon)
2) Remove tampon, give IV fluids, give IV flucloxacillin

QUESTION 46
1) Systemic sclerosis
2) Scl-70 autoantibodies may be positive
3) Renal hypertensive crisis and pulmonary fibrosis

QUESTION 47
1) Renal cell carcinoma
2) CT or U/S abdomen

QUESTION 48
1) Myotonic dystrophy

QUESTION 49
1) Hypothyroidism
2) Obstructive sleep apnoea
3) TSH, polysomnography studies

QUESTION 50
1) *Legionella* pneumonia
2) Macrolides (e.g. erythromycin) or tetracyclines

QUESTION 51
1) Gitelman's syndrome
2) Potassium supplements, NSAIDs

QUESTION 52
1) Myelodysplasia
2) Bone marrow aspiration and trephine

QUESTION 53
1) Pregnancy
2) Referral to GP or obstetrician for continued care

QUESTION 54
Friedreich's ataxia

QUESTION 55
1) Weil's disease
2) Blood cultures, CSF culture

QUESTION 56
1) Haemochromatosis
2) Liver biopsy for iron studies

QUESTION 57
1) Tuberculosis
2) Flexible bronchoscopy with alveolar lavage for culture of *Mycobacterium tuberculosis* and tuberculin test
3) Chest drain for the pneumothorax and triple therapy with isoniazid, pyrazinamide and rifampicin

QUESTION 58
1) Relapsing polychondritis
2) Nasal cartilage biopsy

QUESTION 59
1) Eclampsia with DIC and renal impairment
2) Control of blood pressure with IV hydralazine, control of fitting with magnesium sulphate, delivery of baby

QUESTION 60
1) Phenytoin toxicity
2) Phenytoin levels
3) Stop phenytoin, and reintroduce at lower dose later with level monitoring

QUESTION 61
1) Alpha-1-antitrypsin deficiency
2) Serum electrophoresis to look for $\alpha 1 AT$ isomers

QUESTION 62
1) Addison's disease
2) Short synacthen test, ACTH levels, adrenal autoantibodies

QUESTION 63
1) Iron deficiency anaemia, thalassaemia
2) Hb electrophoresis, iron studies

QUESTION 64
1) Falciparum malaria
2) Thick and thin blood films, urine microscopy and culture, blood glucose
3) Quinine

QUESTION 65
1) Autoimmune polyglandular syndrome type 2 (Addison's, hypothyroidism and diabetes)
2) Thyroid function tests, short synacthen test

QUESTION 66
1) Ebstein's anomaly with WPW
2) Echocardiogram

QUESTION 67
1) Multiple myeloma leading to a vertebral wedge fracture
2) Bone marrow biopsy, urinalysis for Bence-Jones proteins, skeletal survey, serum electrophoresis with Ig quantification

QUESTION 68
1) Budd-Chiari syndrome
2) Liver ultrasound with Doppler

QUESTION 69
1) Paget's disease of bone
2) Plain radiographs, radioisotope bone scan, urine hydroxyproline levels

QUESTION 70
1) TTP
2) Eclampsia, HUS, SLE
3) Gum biopsy

QUESTION 71
1) Addisonian crisis
2) Intravenous hydrocortisone
3) Blood glucose, MRI pituitary fossa, morning serum cortisol, serum prolactin, testosterone ACTH levels

QUESTION 72
1) Mixed essential cryoglobulinaemia
2) Cryoglobulins, hepatitis C serology

QUESTION 73
1) Wegener's granulomatosis
2) Renal biopsy, cANCA, anti-GBM antibodies to exclude Goodpasture's syndrome

QUESTION 74
1) Carbon monoxide poisoning

QUESTION 75
1) Acromegaly
2) MRI of the pituitary

QUESTION 76
1) Hypogammaglobulinaemia
2) Immunoglobulin subclass analysis, chest X-ray, sigmoidoscopy, barium enema

QUESTION 77
1) Ventricular tachycardia due to digoxin toxicity because of raised levels from the erythromycin
2) Digoxin levels
3) Digoxin-specific antibody fragments and withdrawal of digoxin

QUESTION 78
1) Syphilis
2) Serology with TPHA
3) HIV infection
4) Procaine penicillin

QUESTION 79
1) Paroxysmal nocturnal haemoglobinuria with DVT
2) Urine microscopy, Ham's test and U/S or venography of the left leg

QUESTION 80
1) Giant cell arteritis
2) High dose prednisolone

QUESTION 81
1) Optic neuritis secondary to multiple sclerosis
2) MRI brain, CSF analysis for protein, immunoglobulins and lymphocytes compared with blood and visual and auditory evoked potentials
3) High dose oral steroids

QUESTION 82
1) Bacterial overgrowth, short bowel syndrome, active Crohn's disease, infective colitis, e.g. pseudomembranous colitis
2) Stool for microscopy, culture and *Clostridium difficile* toxin, plain abdominal X-ray to exclude toxic megacolon

QUESTION 83
1) Botulism
2) Mouse bioassay for toxins

3) Mechanical ventilation, IV fluids, antitoxin against botulinum toxins

QUESTION 84
1) SLE
2) DVT secondary to antiphospholipid syndrome
3) dsDNA, ANA, anticardiolipin antibody, renal biopsy

QUESTION 85
1) Rheumatic fever, acute juvenile arthritis
2) Rheumatic fever
3) Bed rest, aspirin and penicillin

QUESTION 86
1) Ecstasy overdose
2) Hyperpyrexia, shock, renal failure, ARDS, DIC
3) Urine MDMA screen, CK level
4) Intravenous fluids, diazepam, ventilation and intensive monitoring

QUESTION 87
1) This man probably has an HIV related illness – the headache could be due to:
   Cerebral toxoplasmosis
   TB meningitis
   Cryptococcal meningitis
   Lymphoma
   Other aseptic meningitides
2) CT brain with contrast, lumbar puncture, with India Ink and ZN stains, HIV test

QUESTION 88
1) Lithium levels
2) Intravenous fluids. Stop lithium, diuretics, ACE-I
3) Lithium toxicity with renal failure

QUESTION 89
1) PCP, radiation lung fibrosis, bilateral bacterial pneumonia, lymphangitis carcinomatosa
2) Bronchoalveolar lavage with microscopy with silver stain

QUESTION 90
1) Tricyclic antidepressant overdose

QUESTION 91
1) Tuberculosis, bronchial carcinoma, and pulmonary embolism

2) Chest X-ray, bronchoscopy and brushing for cytology and culture including TB culture, sputum for microscopy, culture (including TB) and a CT pulmonary angiogram for PE and malignancy

QUESTION 92
1) Lyme disease
2) Cardiac pacing; may need permanent pacing. IV cephalosporins or penicillin

QUESTION 93
1) Pseudohypoparathyroidism
2) Hand X-rays, Chase-Auerbach test

QUESTION 94
1) Adult onset Still's disease
2) High dose NSAIDs

QUESTION 95
1) Ethylene glycol poisoning
2) Ethylene glycol levels, urinalysis for oxalate crystals, blood lactate
3) Ethanol, followed by dialysis

QUESTION 96
1) Myasthenia gravis
2) Guillain-Barré syndrome
3) Anti ACh receptor antibodies, Tensilon test, vital capacity

QUESTION 97
1) Acute autoimmune hepatitis leading to hepatic failure

QUESTION 98
1) Amyloidosis secondary to rheumatoid arthritis
2) Rectal or renal biopsy

QUESTION 99
1) Antiphospholipid syndrome
2) Anticardiolipin antibodies, or failure of APTT to correct with addition of normal plasma

QUESTION 100
1) Brucellosis
2) Lymphoma, CLL, CML
3) Bone marrow biopsy, blood cultures, *Brucella* serology

NORMAL VALUES

14

BIOCHEMISTRY

Na 136–149 mmol/L
K 3.8–5.0 mmol/L
Urea 2.5–6.5 mmol/L
Creatinine 55–125 μmol/L
Total protein 65–80 g/L
Albumin 35–55 g/L
Bilirubin 2–13 μmol/L
ALT 5–27 iu/L
ALP 30–130 iu/L
Gamma GT 0–30 iu/L
Chloride 93–108 mmol/L
Bicarbonate 24–30 mmol/L
Calcium 2.15–2.65 mmol/L
Phosphate 0.8–1.4 mmol/L
Uric acid 0.1–0.4 mmol/L
CK 0–170 iu/L
Plasma osmolality 285–295 mosmol/kg
Cholesterol 3.6–5.0 mmol/L
Triglyceride 0–2.0 mmol/L
Glucose 3.5–5.5 mmol/L
IgG 5–16 g/L
IgA 1.25–4.25 g/L
IgM 0.5–1.7 g/L
CRP 0–10 mg/L
Iron 16–30 μmol/L (males)
Iron 11–27 μmol/L (females)
TIBC 45–72 μmol/L
Vit B_{12} 200–900 pg/L
Mg 0.65–1 mmol/L
Faecal fat excretion <6 g/24 h
PSA 0–6 mg/L
Vitamin D 15–100 mmol/L

HORMONES

Cortisol 170–720 nmol/L (9 a.m.)
Cortisol 170–220 nmol/L (midnight)

Growth hormone <10 ng/mL
Thyroxine 70–160 nmol/L
TSH 0.8–3.6 mU/L

HAEMATOLOGY

Hb 13.5–17.5 g/dL (males)
Hb 11.5–15.5 g/dL (females)
MCH 27–32 pg
MCHC 32–36 g/dL
MCV 76–98 fl
Reticulocyte count 0.2–2%
Platelet count 150–400 × 10^9/L
WCC 4–11 × 10^9/L
Neutrophils 2.5–7.5 × 10^9/L
Lymphocytes 1.5–3.5 × 10^9/L
Eosinophils 0.04–0.44 × 10^9/L
Basophils 0–0.1 × 10^9/L
Monocytes 0.2–0.8 × 10^9/L
ESR 0–10 mm/h
Prothrombin time 12–15.5 s
Activated partial thromboplastin time 30–46 s
Thrombin time 15–19 s
Bleeding time 2–8 min
Fibrinogen 2–4 g/L

CARDIOLOGY

RA 4 mmHg (3.2–4.8)
RV (end diastole) 4 (mean) mmHg
RV (systole) 25 (mean), (range 15–30) mmHg
PA (diastole) 10 (mean), (range 5–15) mmHg
PA (systole) 25 (mean), (range 5–30) mmHg
PAWP 10 (mean), (range 5–14) mmHg
LV (end diastole) 7 (mean), (range 4–12) mmHg
LV (systole) 120 (mean), (range 100–140) mmHg
Aorta (diastole) 70 (mean), (range 60–90) mmHg
Aorta (systole) 120 (mean), (range 90–140) mmHg

INDEX

Pagination in **bold** indicates a main diagnosis, in *italic* a differential diagnosis. Pagination for the question and answer sections is prefixed by the Q or A number in brackets. Abbreviations are noted but not cross-referenced. For a list of abbreviations see pp. 228–30.